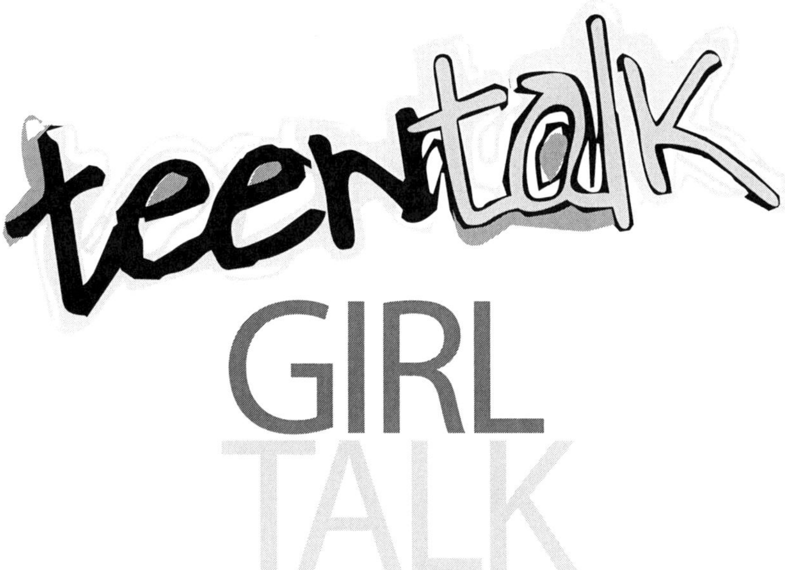

by

Sharon Witt

Important note: The information contained in this book is for educational purposes and should not substitute medical and/ or professional advice, or personal judgement. The author and publisher accept no responsibility for any action taken as a result of this material.

Teen Talk – Girl Talk
Book 2 of the 'Teen Talk' series
Revised and updated edition

Collective Wisdom Publications Pty Ltd
PO Box 150
Mt Evelyn VIC 3796
www.sharonwitt.com.au

First published November 2023
Reprinted May 2024

ISBN: 9780648951759

Requests for information should be addressed to Sharon Witt
sharon@sharonwitt.com.au

Typesetting and design by Communique Graphics
Illustrations by Ivan Smith www.ivansmithdesign.com
Printed in Australia by Openbook Howden Print & Design
www.openbookhowden.com.au
Distributed in Australia by Woodslane Pty Ltd www.woodslane.com.au

THIS BOOK BELONGS TO AN

AMAZING GIRL

____

To my girls

Emi, Em & Maddy

HELLO teen girl

I'm so glad you're here

Hello amazing teen girl,

Welcome to Girl Talk! This is the fully revised and updated version of this book that was first published over 17 years ago! Whilst a great deal has changed in girl world over the past nearly 2 decades, some topics remain mostly unchanged. Girls still experience issues with friendships, body image, and self-esteem. And since the first edition of this book was published, we now have social media to contend with.

If you've picked up this book, or been given it, chances are you're already a teenager, and right in the thick of all the emotional ups and downs, and physical changes. You may feel like your body has been taken over by an alien – your body is doing many new and amazing things (many of which you are totally unaware of!)

Let me assure you of two very important things:

1. You are not alone. Many hundreds of thousands of teen girls all around the world are, right at this very moment, going through similar changes, emotions, and feelings. Girls just like you have similar questions, thoughts, and experiences. You will most likely find the questions throughout this book helpful. They were written by teenage girls just like you (not made up by adults or me!)

2. Everything you are experiencing right now or are soon to experience is **PERFECTLY NORMAL!** Though, at times, navigating the changes of puberty can be a bit scary and unfamiliar, rest assured that all that you feel is right on the scale of normal and you will come through the other side OKAY. ☺

>>>

Just remember, you are an incredible girl in an exciting time of your life. Try and take each day as it comes and do not worry too much (often easier said than done, I know!)

My sincerest hope for you is that this book, written especially for you, will help guide you through this incredible time.

With love,

Sharon x

WHAT'S INSIDE

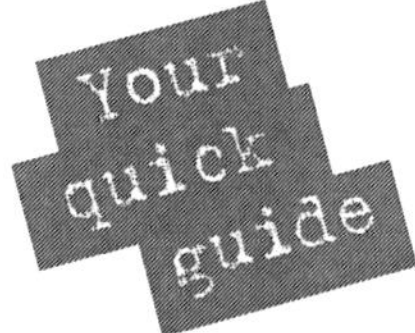

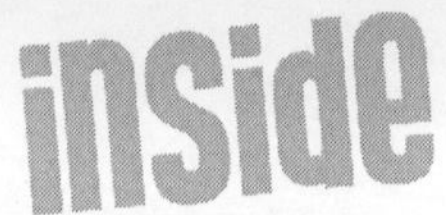

one//

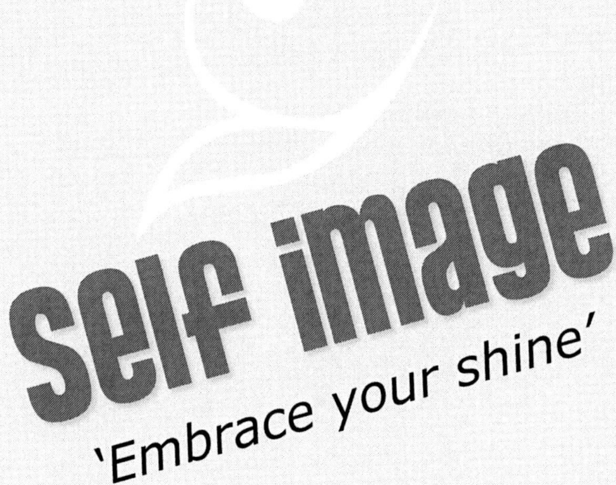

"The most beautiful thing you can wear is confidence."

Blake Lively

being a girl is great!

Being a teen girl is an exciting phase of life that comes with its own set of unique and wonderful experiences. Whilst it's important to acknowledge the challenges you'll experience at this stage, there are many reasons why being a teen girl is great. From self-discovery to personal growth and building strong connections, this period of life offers numerous opportunities for growth and personal development.

During your teen years, you'll begin to explore new interests, passions, and values. This is a time when you can experiment with various hobbies, extracurricular activities, and interests to figure out what truly resonates with you. Whether it's discovering a talent for painting, a passion for writing, or an enthusiasm for science, this time self-exploration allows you to start building the foundation for your future.

You'll have more opportunities to embrace the power of friendship and building meaningful relationships. Girls often form close bonds during these years with their peers that can last a lifetime. The friendships established during this period are characterised by shared experiences, trust, and mutual support.

Your teen years can offer a profound sense of personal growth and development. As you navigate the challenges of adolescence, you'll learn valuable life skills such as problem-solving, decision-making, and responsibility. These experiences will help shape you into a resilient, capable young lady.

Self-esteem

- know your worth!

I want you to know that you are incredible just the way you are. Self-esteem is all about recognising your worth and believing in yourself, and it's a journey that can lead to a happier, more fulfilling life.

quote

'Always be a first-rate version of yourself, instead of a second-rate version of somebody else.'

Judy Garland

First and foremost, remember that you are unique. No one else in this world is exactly like you, and that is your superpower. Embrace your individuality, your quirks, and your flaws. They make you who you are, and that's something to be proud of.

Self-esteem isn't about being perfect; it's about being confident in your imperfections. We all make mistakes and face challenges, but these are opportunities for growth and learning. Don't be too hard on yourself when things don't go as planned. Instead, focus on what you've learned and how you can improve.

"A healthy self-esteem — feeling good about yourself — will reflect on and translate to other people around you."

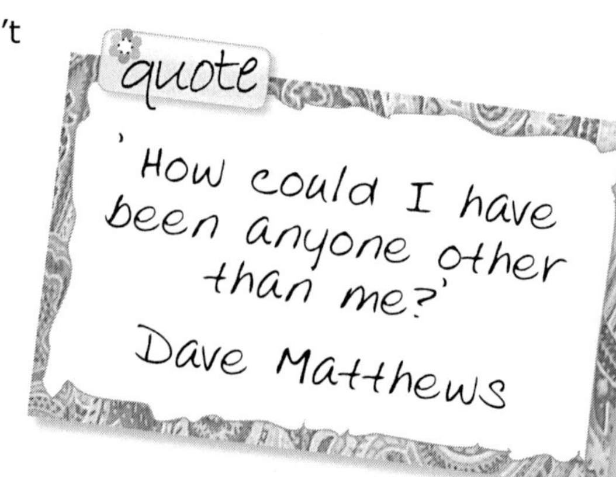

poem

'And so I sit and wait for the day,
When I can be seen in my own special way.
Just myself, how should I be?
Not at all perfect-
Just perfectly me.'

Melissa Munro

quote

'Be yourself.
Nobody is better qualified.'

Anonymous

Developing a healthy self image is one of the most important goals you can concentrate on right now. With a healthy self image, you can accomplish anything you set your mind to!

quote

'If I try to be like him,
who will be like me?'

Jewish Proverb

If you can do all that you can to work on your self image as a teenager, you stand a much greater chance of becoming a happy and successful adult!

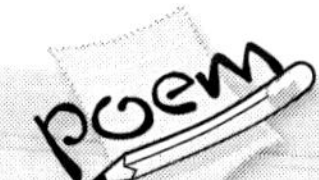

poem

Life, Love & Longing

By Riana Baensch

The breath of life touches my lips
And I come alive to a world of wonders
Love is everywhere but cannot be given
Until you love yourself.
I am no longer in need of acceptance
For I am loved, can love and will love
Until His hand rests upon my shoulder and says that
It is time.

believe in your WORTH

By 'Sally', aged 13

All through Primary School I was bullied for being fat, ugly, geeky — you name it; I was called it!

So after about one year, that's how I began to see myself and I couldn't change my opinion from what was said.

It just stuck.

When I began High School, I had no self-worth or self-esteem — I just wished I wasn't alive. I got really depressed and began to think a lot about suicide and self-harm.

Whenever someone called me beautiful, I always dismissed it as stupid and them just pitying me.

Now that I am in my second year of High School and have heard what those sort of feelings could do to a person, I began talking to people about how I was feeling, asking for advice and support.

It's made me think about a lot of things that I've done to myself.

Hearing stories and advice from my teachers really changed a lot of the ways I'm thinking about my own appearance and self-worth.

Each girl is a princess at heart and she just needs someone to believe in her to say she is worthy.

quote

'Low self-esteem is like driving through life with your handbrake on.'

Maxwell Maltz (1899-1975)
American Surgeon
& motivational writer

feeling more BEAUTIFUL than ever before

By 'Jess', aged 14

When I was younger, I had braces, glasses, a hearing aid (that I thankfully do not need any more!) and I was overweight!

My self-esteem was really low.

Even when I ditched my hearing aid, my braces were taken off and I got contact lenses, I still felt ugly.

But I'm now feeling more beautiful than I've ever felt.

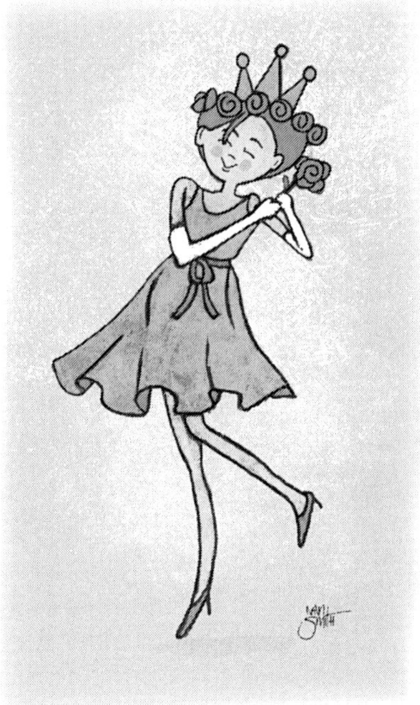

I now know to think more about the things I'm good at rather than the things I don't like about myself.

If I continue to do this, I think I will push all the negativity out and the others will see that too. Then I can help others with low self-esteem to think more positively about themselves!

embrace your Uniqueness

You have been created as a unique and amazing girl, capable of anything! You are truly gorgeous, and you need to hold on to this truth for the rest of your life, no matter what others may say to you or any negative experiences you have. Your uniqueness is what makes you so special. Imagine how boring it would be if everyone was exactly the same. Celebrate the things that are different about you. Be thankful you have crazy freckles or red curly hair. These qualities are the things that make you ***you***!

quote

'If everyone lit their own candle, the whole world would be lit.'

Mary Moskovitz

There were two versions of me at one stage when I was growing up, all because of a TV show called *A Country Practice*. And leading the way was one of the stars, 'Molly'. She was a confident, gorgeous woman who stood up for what she believed in. She dressed in bright colours and wore amazing, wacky, bright outfits. Molly, the character, eventually died. That episode was watched by millions of Australians, sitting glued to their TVs to watch a most-loved character fade from our screens for eternity.

In front of one TV screen was me, crying, tears rolling down, thinking how much I wanted to be 'Molly'.

The truth is, there is only one *you* on the whole face of the earth — how incredible is that!? Being created as a unique and amazing individual actually lets you off the hook straight away. You don't have to try and be anybody else but yourself.

quote

'All of us are stars and deserve the right to twinkle.'

Marilyn Monroe

Actress Judy Garland — the girl who played Dorothy in *The Wizard of Oz* — once said:

> ***'Always be a first-rate version of yourself, instead of a second-rate version of someone else.'***

The media constantly bombards us with images, telling us what we should look like and how we should act as teenagers. We end up becoming lookalikes of each other. How boring is that?

That girl I loved on TV — Molly — affected my dress sense, big time! I remember conning my Nanna into making me a copy of a bright jumpsuit that Molly wore. I even put 'Molly's' bright clips in my hair. (The mental images frighten me to this day!)

quote

'Our problem is that we make the mistake of comparing ourselves with other people. You are not inferior or superior to any human being... You do not determine your success by comparing yourself to others. Rather, you determine your success by comparing your accomplishments to your capabilities. You are "number one" when you do the best you can with what you have, every day.'

Zig Ziglar, American motivational writer

Sure, I went around dressed as 'Molly' for a while, but it wasn't the real me. I was just trying to copy somebody else I admired.

Trends and fashions may come and go, but don't just buy something or wear an outfit because you are trying to be something you are not. You just end up being very uncomfortable because you're not being real to yourself.

you are a Star!

You are a shining star

Precious
Designed intentionally
Wonderfully made

You make this world a better place

You are unavoidably beautiful

Invaluable
Unique
Unlimited in potential

And in you are treasures beyond measure.

Be strong and brave

Dare to be
Realise your beauty
Believe in who you are

Because you are amazing!

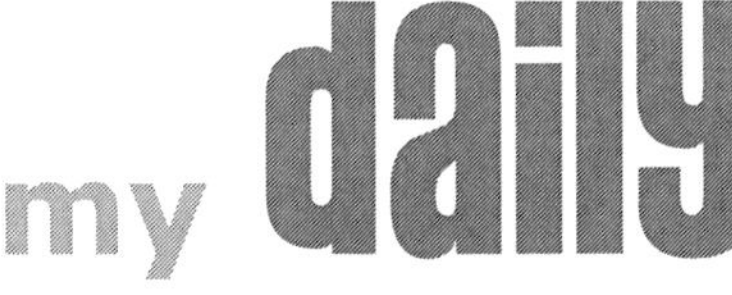

my daily self-evaluation

By Jenny Sharaf

I stare in the mirror,
Pinching the skin around
my stomach,
Moulding it into the
ideal shape.

I wish that I could
look like her,
The girl in the magazine.
I compare our hair and teeth,
Our skin and our lips.

With every look my
self-esteem vanishes.
Losing confidence,
my smile soon fades.
My flaws seem endless and numbered
As I quickly fall into a state of sadness,
And put on a baggy sweatshirt,
Concealing my imperfect figure,
Letting go of my dreams
and pretending I don't care.

Slowly and realistically I begin to accept
My image and identity, repeating to myself
That I am the only me, and that is a good thing.[1]

1 From *No Body's Perfect* by Kimberly Kirberger.
Copyright © 2003 by Kimberly Kirberger. Reprinted by permission of Scholastic Inc.

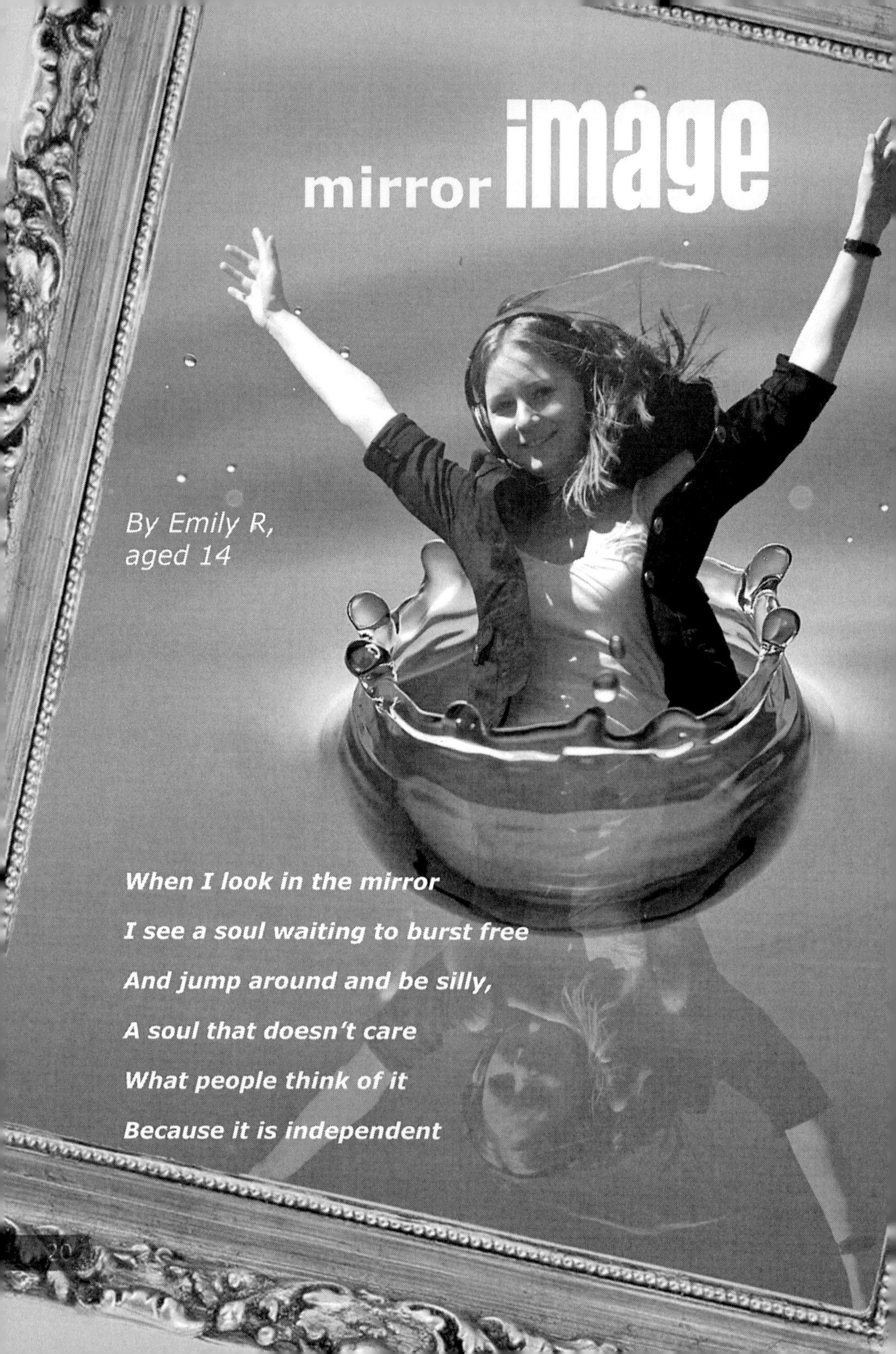

mirror image

By Emily R, aged 14

When I look in the mirror
I see a soul waiting to burst free
And jump around and be silly,
A soul that doesn't care
What people think of it
Because it is independent

when she LOOKS in the mirror

By Taylor D, aged 14

When she looks in the mirror
She sees a girl changing
A girl who has a great chance
To change her life as well.
Chances to let her colours burst out
And show how metallic she really is.

When she looks in the mirror
She sees someone
Who in the past might have
been hiding something
Her true self!

Every day this girl would look
in the mirror
And see only negative things
about herself.
Every day she pretended to
be someone she wasn't
Trying to be noticed and popular.

Then one day this girl looked
in the mirror
And saw her true self
Laughing and having a great time.
And so the next morning
she let her colours show
And funnily enough
She came back from school that day
With nothing but positive thoughts!

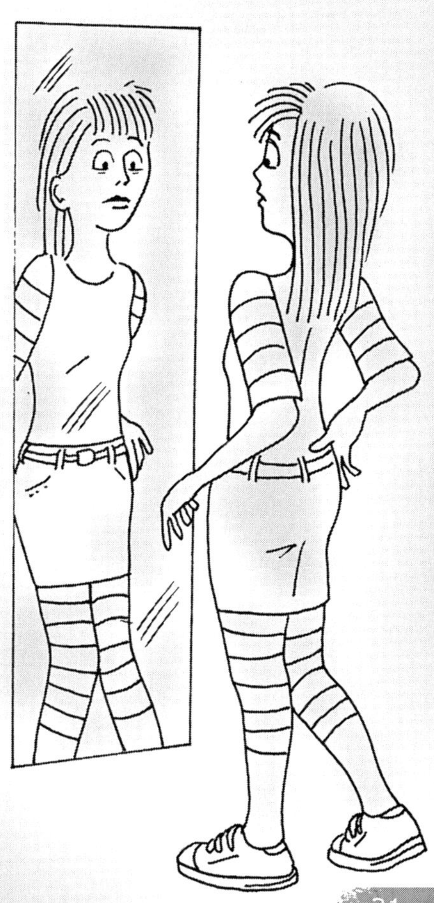

on the inside...

By Emma T, aged 14

Sure, people can be really pretty on the outside,
But on the inside
They could be really mean or not nice at all.

Someone once gave me an example and it goes a bit like this:

You can pick up an apple
and it can look really juicy and tasty
Then you take a bite out of it and it could be
The worst apple you have ever tasted.
It could be rotten and disgusting!

I think that's like people.
You see them at a glance
But it's not until you actually get to know them
That you know what type of person they are.

I think by saying 'on the inside'
A person means that it is what is in one's soul and heart
That is what matters most, and
Who you are as a person.

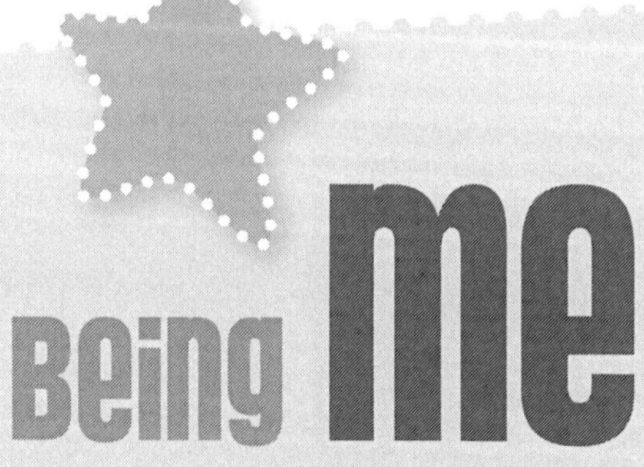

I have a quiz, and as a part of one of the questions it says:
'You never know what's going on behind that perfect facade'.
For example, someone could be really pretty
But could have heaps of problems going on in their lives,
Like family problems, issues with friends,
And lots more.

It's not about outer beauty
It's about inner beauty!

Everyone else was pretty.
I wanted to be the same.
But soon I learnt,
I was taught,
In myself
I should have no shame.

We are all special
In our own very special way,
Nobody can change this
No matter what they say.

[1] Used with permission.

Why can't I be me?
Why does no one see
What I want to be
I just want to be me
If I can't be myself
I'll just be someone else

Anonymous

'I wear glasses and braces and feel like such a nerd. What should I do?'

Ah yes, the nerdy faze! Let me reassure you here that most of us go through a time during our adolescent years when we wish we could be locked in a small, dark, room for a few years until we emerge as a gorgeous, fully grown 18 or 19 year-old — a bit like the story of *The Very Hungry Caterpillar*.

My 'nerd years' involved very scary perms and red rimmed glasses. Yours may involve braces, bad hair cuts or dorky looking glasses. If you didn't go through the pain and inconvenience of braces, you just might be a grown adult with bad eyes and shocking buck teeth! Have you ever seen the 'before' and 'after' photos of celebrities in magazines when they were in college or high school — long before they became famous and had access to hair stylists and makeup artists? They often looked strange and dorky when they were teens too, complete with frizzy hair and braces. You would hardly recognise them as the glamorous and beautiful people they appear to be today.

The thing is, we all go through changes and evolutions, just like a caterpillar! One day, your braces will come off and you will get some trendy glasses or contact lenses. You won't always feel like a nerd, trust me. Many people (including me) want to burn the photos of themselves as teenagers. But someday, those photos will be a wonderful reminder of the beautiful and confident lady you have grown into!

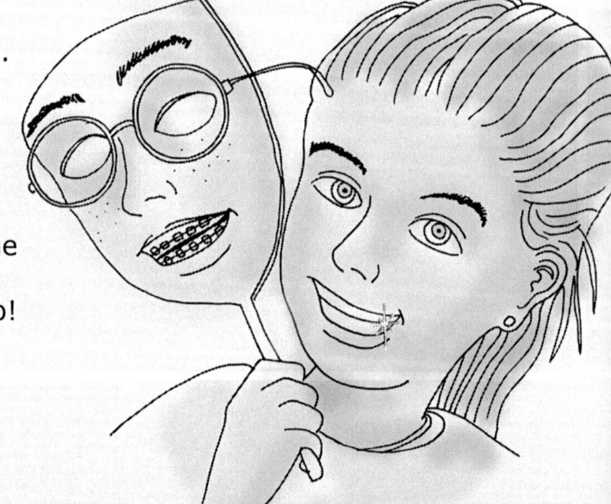

makeUP

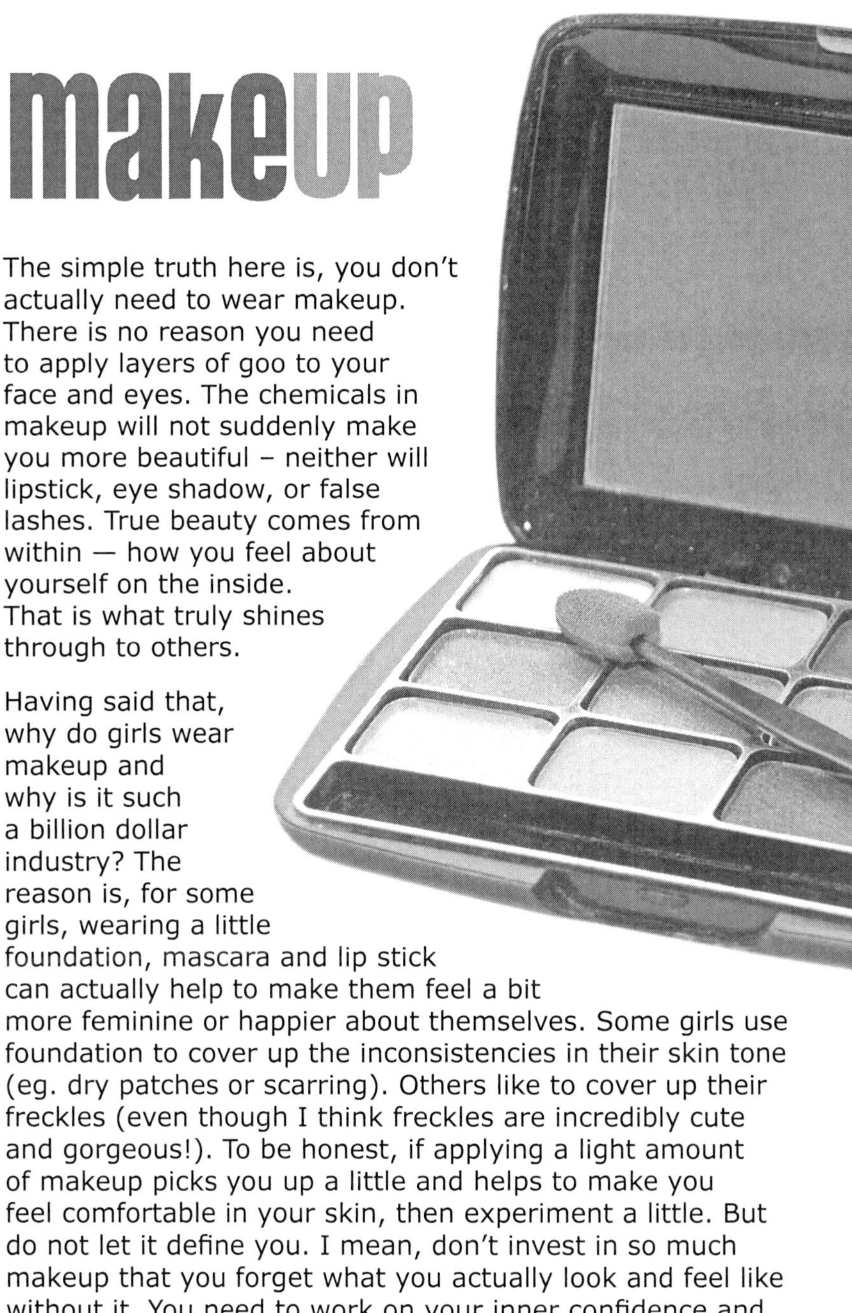

The simple truth here is, you don't actually need to wear makeup. There is no reason you need to apply layers of goo to your face and eyes. The chemicals in makeup will not suddenly make you more beautiful – neither will lipstick, eye shadow, or false lashes. True beauty comes from within — how you feel about yourself on the inside. That is what truly shines through to others.

Having said that, why do girls wear makeup and why is it such a billion dollar industry? The reason is, for some girls, wearing a little foundation, mascara and lip stick can actually help to make them feel a bit more feminine or happier about themselves. Some girls use foundation to cover up the inconsistencies in their skin tone (eg. dry patches or scarring). Others like to cover up their freckles (even though I think freckles are incredibly cute and gorgeous!). To be honest, if applying a light amount of makeup picks you up a little and helps to make you feel comfortable in your skin, then experiment a little. But do not let it define you. I mean, don't invest in so much makeup that you forget what you actually look and feel like without it. You need to work on your inner confidence and self-esteem first. If a little makeup helps you feel better >>>

about yourself, then great, but you shouldn't develop such a habit where you wouldn't want to be seen without it.

The late Princess Diana was known across the world for her beauty and model good looks. Yet I once read a story of her describing how she applied a fresh coat of mascara before she went to bed each evening. When staff enquired as to why she would do such a thing, she replied that it was in case of a fire or emergency and she didn't want to be seen without her mascara on in the middle of the night!

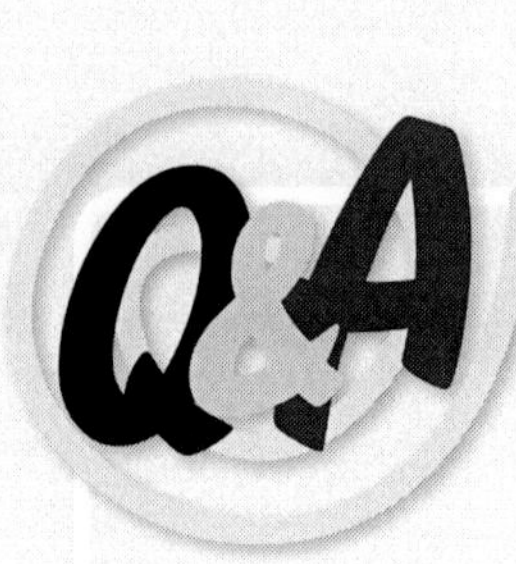

At what age should I start wearing makeup?

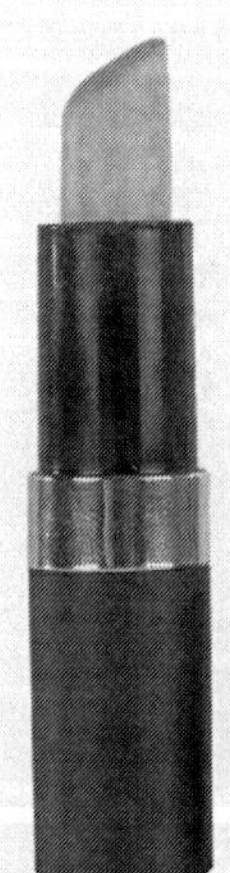

There's no right or wrong answer here, but I would suggest you do not start wearing makeup in primary school. Seek guidance from your parents on this one! Experimenting with makeup during your teen years is fairly common amongst most girls. Perhaps for a special occasion or a family wedding you could ask mum or your caregiver to let you have a turn at using some of her makeup.

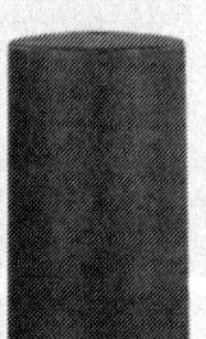

Having someone guiding you is a helpful thing — sometimes we can get a little carried away with what we think looks okay.

prettier without

Emma, aged 14

Makeup makes you feel pretty,
or it covers up all the things that you don't like on your face,
but heaps of people think you look much prettier without it,
especially if it hasn't been done very well.
Just try and stick to a little bit of lip gloss
and a little more makeup for special occasions.
Besides, apart from that,
you look prettier without it.
Things like foundation and other products cover pimples,
and using a lot of eyeliner all the time can cause
black lines under your eyes.

me, not someone else

Jenny, aged 14

I always thought the most important thing was to look nice. My appearance was very important. Having listened to truly beautiful girls saying they were not pretty enough, or wanting to change their body image was upsetting.

I want people to be able to like me as me, not someone else. Sometimes I know that people talk about me — saying what I look like — behind my back, but I have learnt not to worry about what anyone else says but just to know that God loves me more than anyone else will.

Looking 'pretty' may seem like the most important thing but having to change your image just to get people to look at you isn't being yourself.

I want people to be able to like me as me

from the inside out[1]

By Zahava Stadler

I wasn't allowed to wear much makeup. But I thought my skin was uneven and I had circles under my eyes, so I begged my mother for foundation. When she finally caved in, I wore it to school with pride.

A few weeks later, I heard that going to sleep without taking off your foundation would clog your pores. Pimples? I didn't want pimples! So I borrowed my sister's makeup remover towelettes that evening as pre-emptive damage control.

I was astonished to see that at the end of the day, hardly any makeup came off. I wiped harder. Still nothing. Most of the makeup had worn off already. But I still looked good! How could that be?

It was then that I realised that the makeup had given me self-confidence, something I had needed badly. Because of that confidence, even without makeup, I shone from the inside out.

I still wore foundation the next day. But I knew that no matter how uneven my skin tone seemed to me or how tired I looked, when I smiled the smile of pride, confidence or just plain happiness, I would look good. I would be lit up from the inside out.

Feeling good about yourself makes you the most beautiful person alive.

[1] From *No Body's Perfect* by Kimberly Kirberger,

how I see myself

Anonymous, aged 14

I don't think I'm ugly,
        but I don't think I am beautiful.
I have freckles — I absolutely hate them!
They make me feel so ugly sometimes.
All my friends are all pretty
        and look beautiful all the time.
When I am around them
        I feel less important and ugly.
They are really great friends,
        and always include me, which helps heaps!

I spend lots of time in the mornings
        putting foundation on
        to cover up my freckles, bags and pimples.
I go to school in a bad mood
        if I don't like how I look in the mirror
        before I leave.
I mainly do this because
        I like to feel happy and look nice.
I want boys to think I'm pretty
        so they will like me more.
I spend heaps of money on nice clothes
        just so I can look nice for school.

I don't feel beautiful inside,
        because I always compare myself
                to everyone else.

makeup tips!

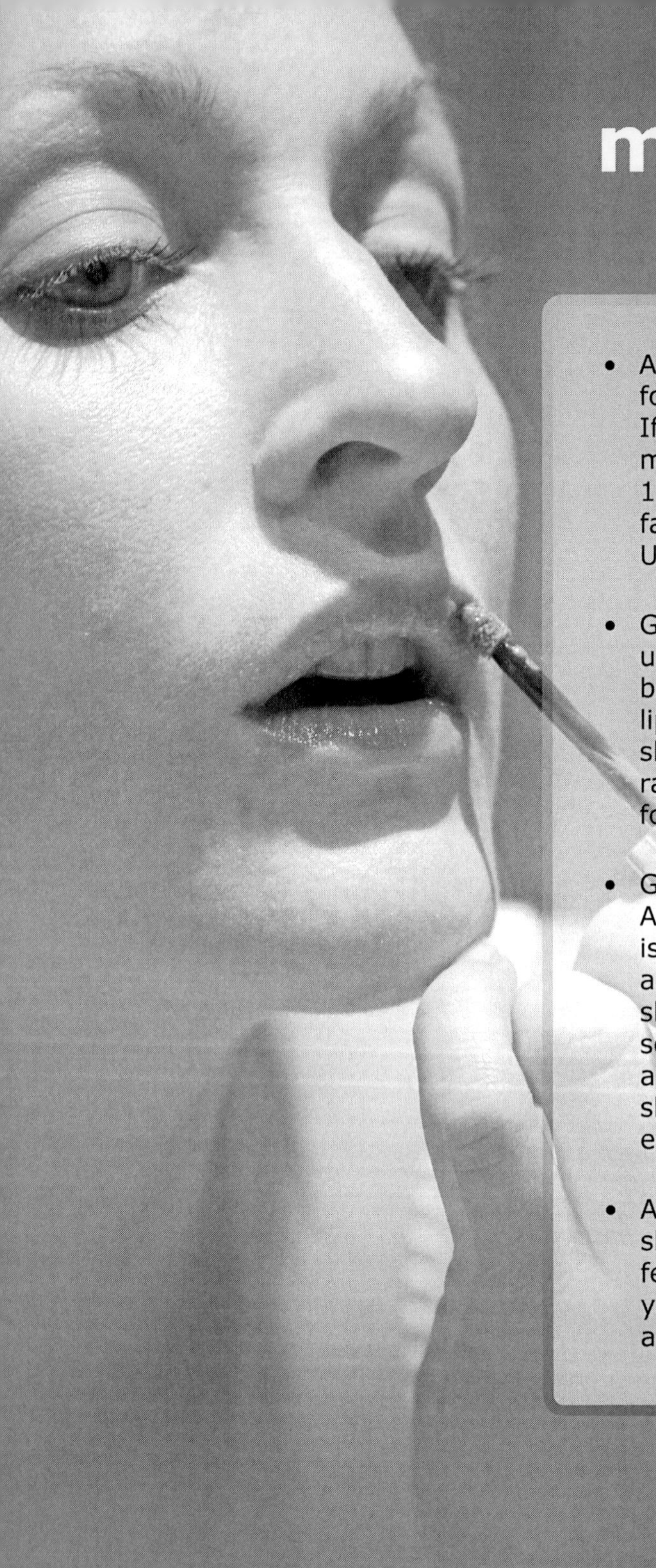

- Apply only a light foundation to your face. If possible, use a tinted moisturiser with SPF 15/30+ to protect your face against the harmful UV rays of the Sun.
- Go easy. Experiment using light shades to begin with. Try a light lip gloss or a light matt shade like a soft pink, rather than going straight for garish bright red.
- Go gently on your eyes. A light level of mascara is a good start. You can add a light amount of eye shadow if you're going somewhere special. As a guide, eye makeup should highlight your eyes.
- Any makeup you use should enhance your features, not transform your face into a work of art.

two//

navigating puberty

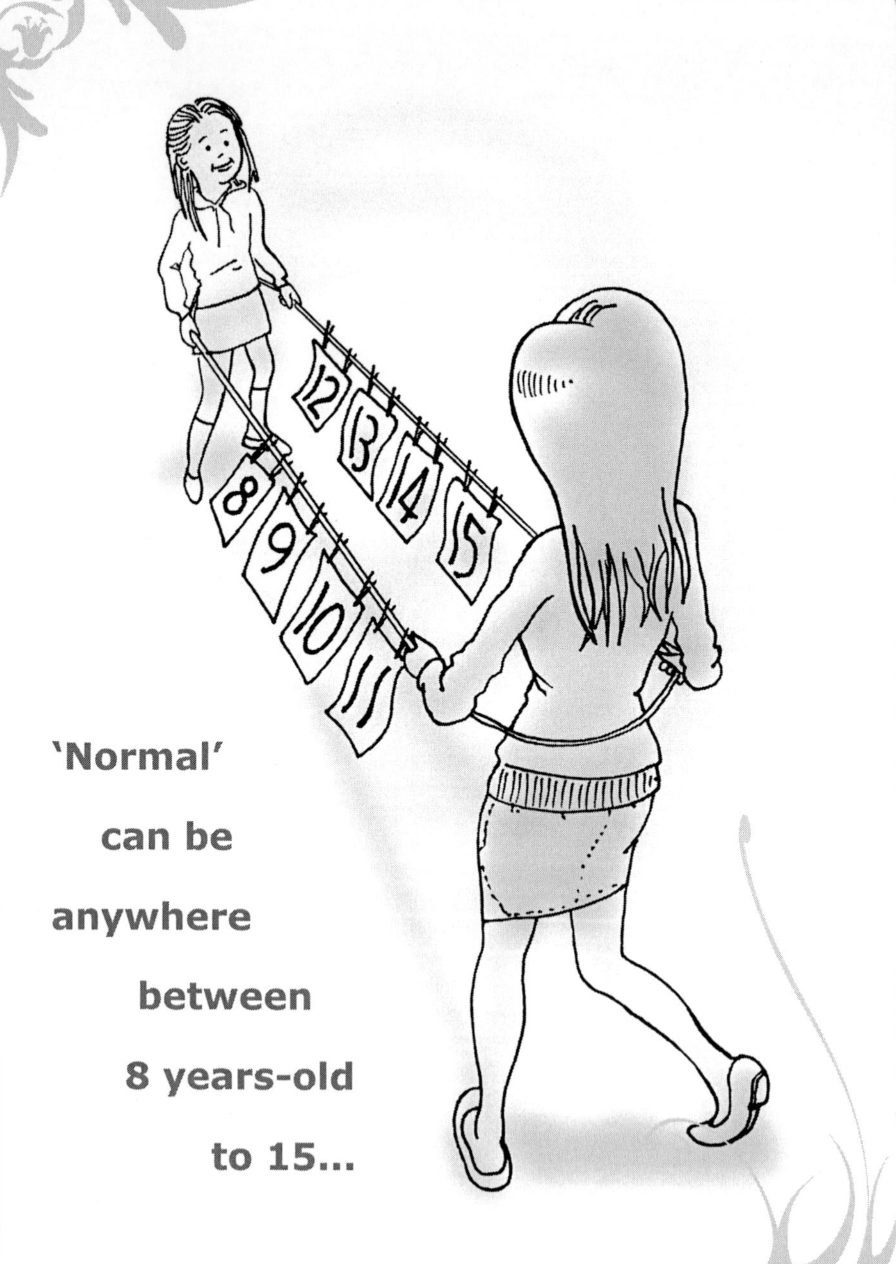

'Normal' can be anywhere between 8 years-old to 15...

when will puberty hit?

I have been teaching young people about puberty for the past thirty years, and by far one of the most common questions asked is – 'When will I start going through puberty?'

The process of Puberty begins when one part of the brain (**the hypothalamus**) communicates with another part of the brain (**the pituitary gland**) to release special hormones. These hormones tell the body to create a special hormone called **Estrogen** in females (for boys, this hormone is known as **Testosterone**).

The simple answer is this – you can't predict when you'll begin the process of your body and mind altering during the puberty phase, however, what I can promise you is it will not all happen in one day! The process of puberty – both the physical and emotional changes, will most likely progress over a few years.

There is no set age that you will notice the changes related to puberty – some girls can notice some small changes as early as eight or nine years old, while others may begin this process when they enter their teenage years. Imagine a long piece of string with a tab for each age from 8 years, right through to 16 years. Girls will typically go through puberty at some stage during that time.

Genetics can also play a part. You may like to ask your mum or another female relative what age they were when they went through puberty. Research has also shown that some girls who are very active or carrying less weight, may go through puberty later, while girls who are extra tall, or carrying extra weight may begin puberty earlier than their peers. I know this doesn't help to pinpoint an exact age, however, it's important for you to know that whatever age this process begins for YOU is perfectly normal.

why do girls go through puberty at different ages??

It has a lot to do with genetics (when your mum, sister or aunty went through puberty) as well as diet and exercise.

Research has shown that some girls who work out and play sport constantly can go through puberty later. Diet is also said to have an impact on when you start puberty.

You need to know that at whatever age it happens for ***you*** is ***perfectly normal***! You also need to be aware that there is nothing at all that you can possibly do to speed up or slow down this process. So you may as well relax and try and enjoy this amazing stage of your life.

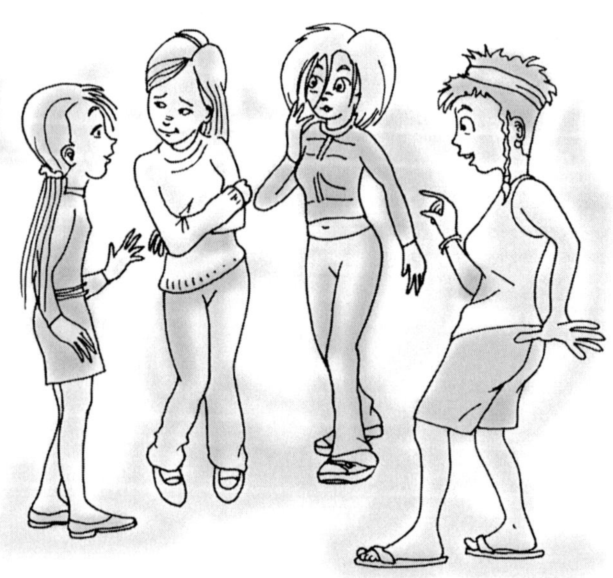

Physical Changes...

- *Breasts begin to develop*
- *Nipples can change size and become darker*
- *Voice can change (deepens — doesn't sound so much like a little girl's anymore!)*
- *Vaginal discharge can increase*
- *Menstruation (periods) begin*
- *Body shape begins to change (hips begin to widen)*
- *Increase in body fat*
- *Pubic hair grows in the genital area and under arms*
- *Skin can change, become oily and pimples may increase due to hormonal changes.*

Parts of a girl's reproductive system

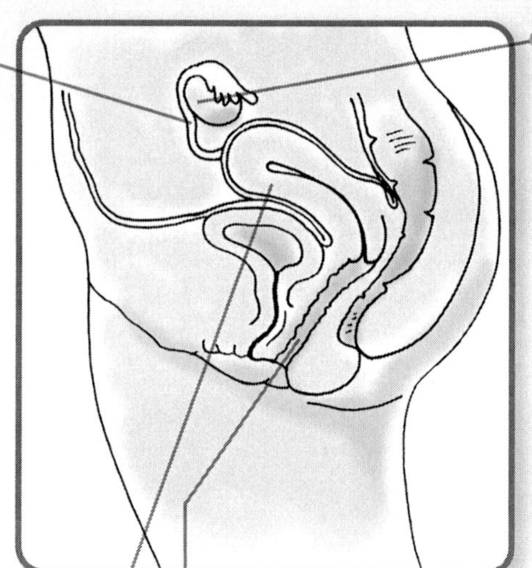

Fallopian tubes

There are two fallopian tubes that join to each side of the uterus or womb. The fallopian tubes are approximately 10cm long and are about the width of spaghetti. When an egg is released from the ovary each month, it travels along the fallopian tube to wait for the possibility of being fertilised by a male sex cell (sperm).

Ovaries

Girls are born with two ovaries (pronounced *ow-ver-ees*), one on either side of the uterus. Each ovary is about 2.5cm long and contains thousands of egg cells capable of being fertilised to develop into a baby.

Once a girl reaches puberty, these ova (eggs) mature and one is released each month from one of the ovaries.

Uterus

The uterus is also known as the womb. It is a hollow, muscly organ that is about the size of a small orange. It sits behind the bladder down low in a girl's abdomen. During a pregnancy, it expands greatly to accommodate the developing baby. After childbirth, it shrinks back down to its original size.

Vagina

The vagina is a muscly tube, about 10cm in length. At the end of the vagina is the cervix, which is the entrance to the uterus or womb. Menstrual blood passes through the vagina during a girl's period. The muscles in the vagina also are able to hold a tampon in place during menstruation if a girl chooses to use one. During child birth, the vagina stretches wide to allow a safe passage for a baby to enter the world.

curves...

When you begin going through puberty, one of the things you may notice is that you will begin to gain weight. It's okay. This is supposed to happen! Your body produces more body fat so that you can develop fuller breasts, hips, stomach and thighs. As your hip bones grow wider (to prepare your body for the possibility of childbirth one day) your waist may appear smaller. These changes help to give your body the shape of a young woman.

Some girls may become concerned that they are putting on weight and changing body shape. It's important to remember that this is ***perfectly normal***! Be careful not to confuse these changes with 'getting fat'.

Gaining weight during puberty is an important part of normal growth and nothing to worry about. You may also notice that as your shape changes, your clothes don't fit the way they used to. For example, you may notice hips widen as your body changes. You no longer have a little girl's body anymore, and that's a great thing. It's supposed to be that way!

If you are concerned about excess weight, please don't worry. Talk to a parent, doctor or school counsellor before you even think of going on a diet. I am sure that they will just reassure you that you are perfect the way you are!

Finally, I know this may be a little difficult, but try not to compare your body to your friend's. Just as every personality is different, so too are our bodies. Absolutely no one will develop in exactly the same way as another and we cannot expect to have the same body type as a friend's. Our genetics determine what type of body we have and you cannot change your body shape. Try to love and accept the body that you have because you are beautiful just as you are!

the breast

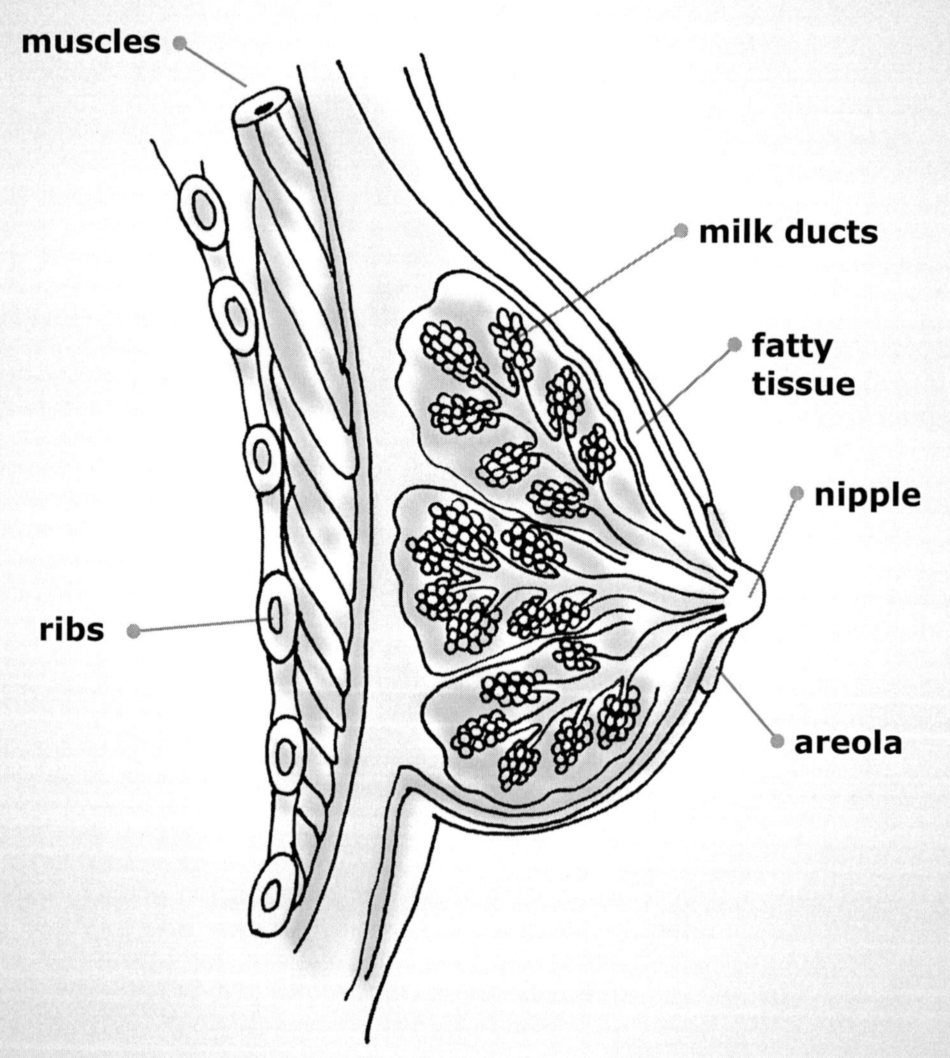

breasts

Breasts (or mammary glands) are one of the more noticeable parts about hitting puberty and becoming a young woman.

The main function and reason behind having breasts in the first place is to prepare a young lady for the possibility of one day having and breast-feeding children of her own. Although this should be a very long way off, you body is developing this equipment for the experience and possibility of childbirth.

Breasts are mostly made up of lumpy, fatty tissue that contains **mammary glands** (the glands that produce milk for a baby). Breasts develop in many different shapes and sizes. Whatever your size, that will be ***normal for you***.

When your breasts first begin to develop, it is normal for them to feel a little strange – like lumpy and bumpy. Your breast development first begins with tiny breast buds that will continue to develop over time. This is all part of the growing process.

When your breasts first begin to develop, it is normal for them to feel a little strange.

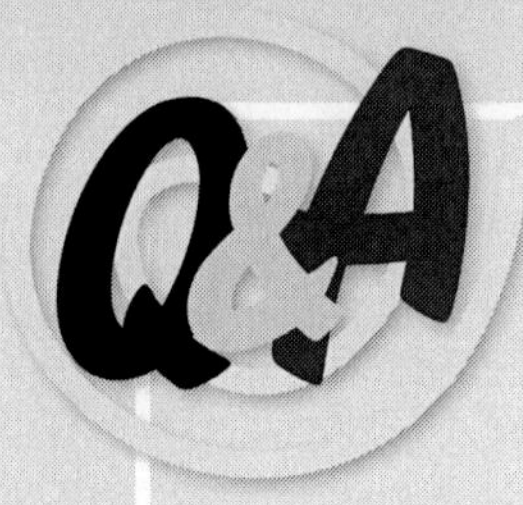

Why do girls have different coloured nipples?

Why are some girls taller than others? Why are some girls blonde, and some brunette? It all comes down to each and every one of us being created as unique and amazing individuals. No two girls will develop at the same pace, or have exactly the same body features, including nipples.

Why do my breasts sometimes feel sore?

During different times of each month, a girl's breasts may feel sore or tender to touch because of hormonal changes. Some girls say their breasts become sore just before they get their period. This can also simply be a sign that your breasts are growing. If you experience any type of severe pain, however, and it happens often, please talk to your trusted adult and they may suggest a check up with your doctor.

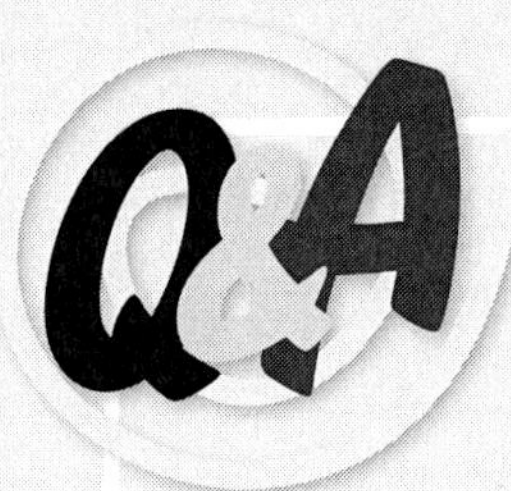

Why are my boobs smaller than most girls my age?

All girls develop at a different stage and pace. How boring would it be if we all were exactly the same? Your breasts may appear smaller than other girls because others may be further developed than you. Or, you may just have a different genetic makeup than who you are comparing yourself to. For example, if your mother has smaller sized breasts, you may experience the same because you share a similar body type. No matter what size breasts you develop, they will work exactly the same way, so try not to worry. Be happy with your body!

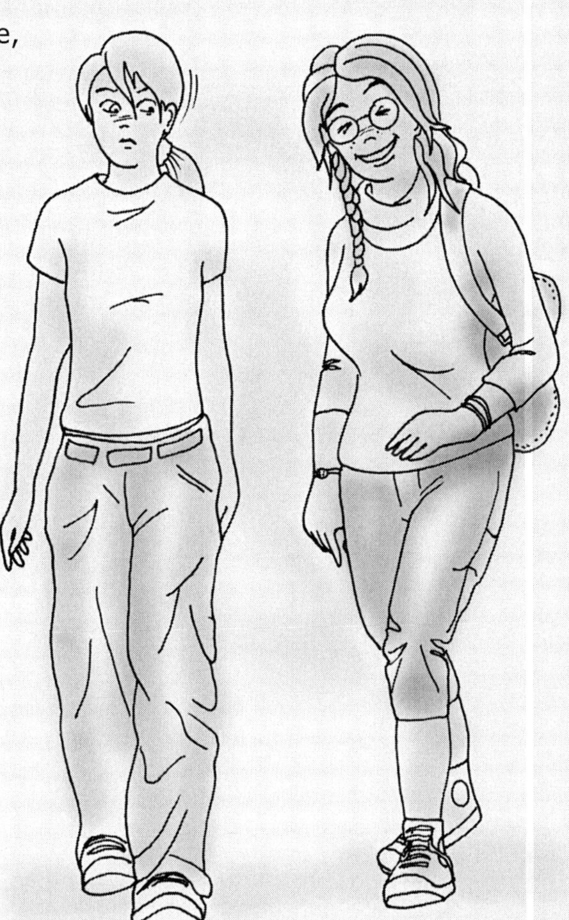

It is quite normal to feel unhappy with your breast size. Girls with larger breasts often complain that they wish they were less heavy and had smaller breasts, whilst those with smaller boobs wish they were a lot bigger.

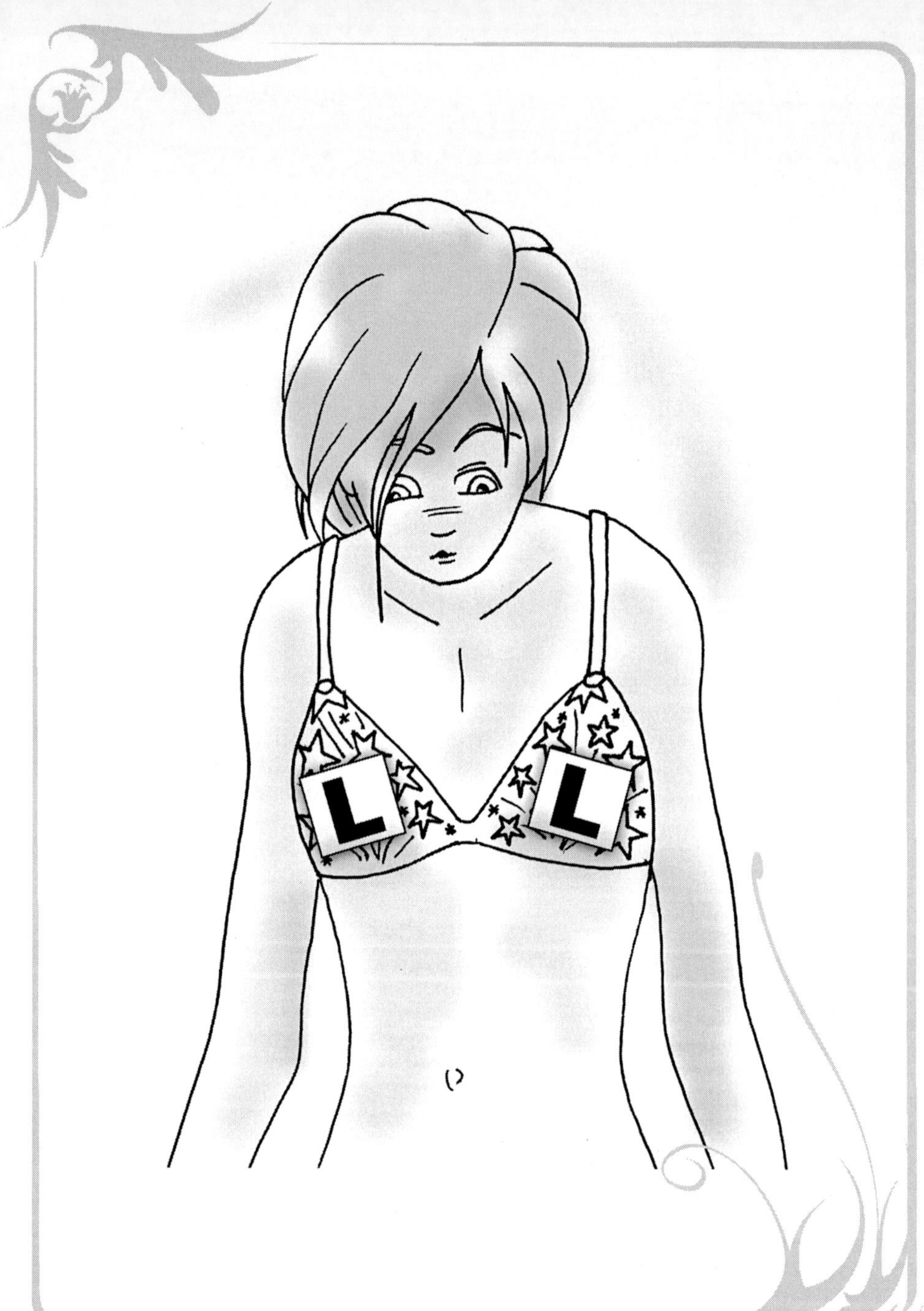
L
L

it's time to buy a bra!

I put off this little excursion for as long as I possibly could...

...because I just couldn't cope with the thought of my mum taking me in to a shop to get fitted for my first bra – I could think of nothing more embarrassing!

Mum would often ask me if it was time we went and bought a bra. I'd run like the wind to avoid that discussion. Eventually, we did venture out and purchase my first little training bra. I survived, although I really did think that absolutely EVERYONE could notice that I was wearing a bra and that it stuck out like a big neon sign on top of my head, flashing ***'Sharon is now wearing a bra!'***

A note of warning here, girls. Don't put off getting fitted for a bra too late. You definitely don't want your boobs sagging down around your belly button when you're an adult.

I really did think that absolutely EVERYONE could notice ... 'Sharon is now wearing a bra!'

'I think I have breast cancer!'

I want to share a very personal experience with you.

Don't laugh! This could be you reading this. Although I am not poking fun at the awful disease that is breast cancer, some girls honestly think that the changes, lumps and bumps they experience are the early signs of breast disease. Let me assure you that it is more than likely you do not have breast cancer, but rather that you're experiencing normal breast development.

When our breasts start to develop they can be quite lumpy – and that can cause anxiety. I actually experienced this fear when I was about 13 years of age. I honestly believed that my normally developing breasts were tumours that would take my life. I always thought that my breasts would be just pillowy-type balloons that didn't really have much substance to them. Then they started to get really lumpy and I just freaked out. I would often lie in bed at night and wonder how much further these cancerous lumps would spread and I would have to tell my parents that I was dying!

Note: *It is important to get your breasts checked out if you feel anything might be abnormal! Whilst it is most likely not cancer, it is always better to get checked than to do nothing. Extra soreness, bleeding or other fluid from the nipples should be particularly checked out. Please make sure that you do this!*

Finally, after probably a year or two, I worked up the courage to break it to my mum that I thought I had breast cancer and I had let it go far too long! With a little smile on her face, she gently reassured me that I probably wasn't dying, but took me to the local doctor anyway, who checked my breasts and assured me that it was normal for my development.

In relaying this little story to a group of my teenage students recently, I wasn't too surprised to hear that others had thought the same thing when they first began getting boobs. So please be assured that all the lumpy and bumpy stuff is perfectly normal.

bra stories...

A collection of memories and anecdotes from girls and women who've survived their bra experiences and seen the lighter side of the dramas...

'I remember I had just brought a new strapless bra and thought I would try it out and wear it to school the next day. Unfortunately, we had Athletics Day (woops) and whenever I ran, the bra just slid off my rather small boobs and settled around my waist. It was quite tricky getting it back up without people realising what I was doing. Eventually I gave up and just sat with my arms over my chest hoping that no one would notice!'

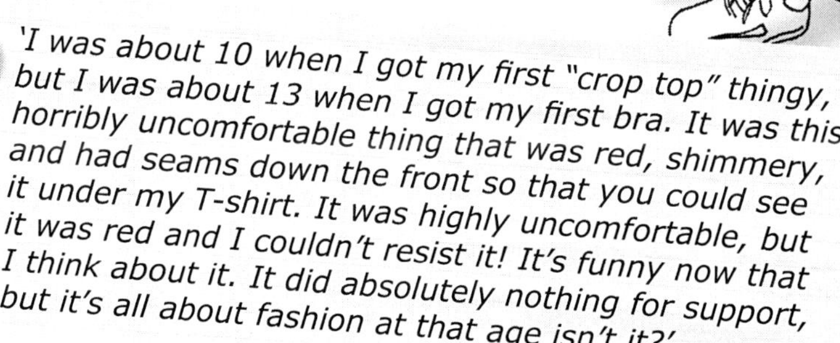

'I was about 10 when I got my first "crop top" thingy, but I was about 13 when I got my first bra. It was this horribly uncomfortable thing that was red, shimmery, and had seams down the front so that you could see it under my T-shirt. It was highly uncomfortable, but it was red and I couldn't resist it! It's funny now that I think about it. It did absolutely nothing for support, but it's all about fashion at that age isn't it?'

'I was as flat as a pancake until the age of 18! But I was so desperate to be like "all the other girls" that my mum bought me one of those flimsy, elastic, do-up-at-the-front type bras when I was 14. Since I couldn't possibly fill the bra with the 'real thing', I had to fill it with tissues. I'm sure that everyone knew that they weren't the 'real deal', but I didn't care. I was wearing my first bra!'

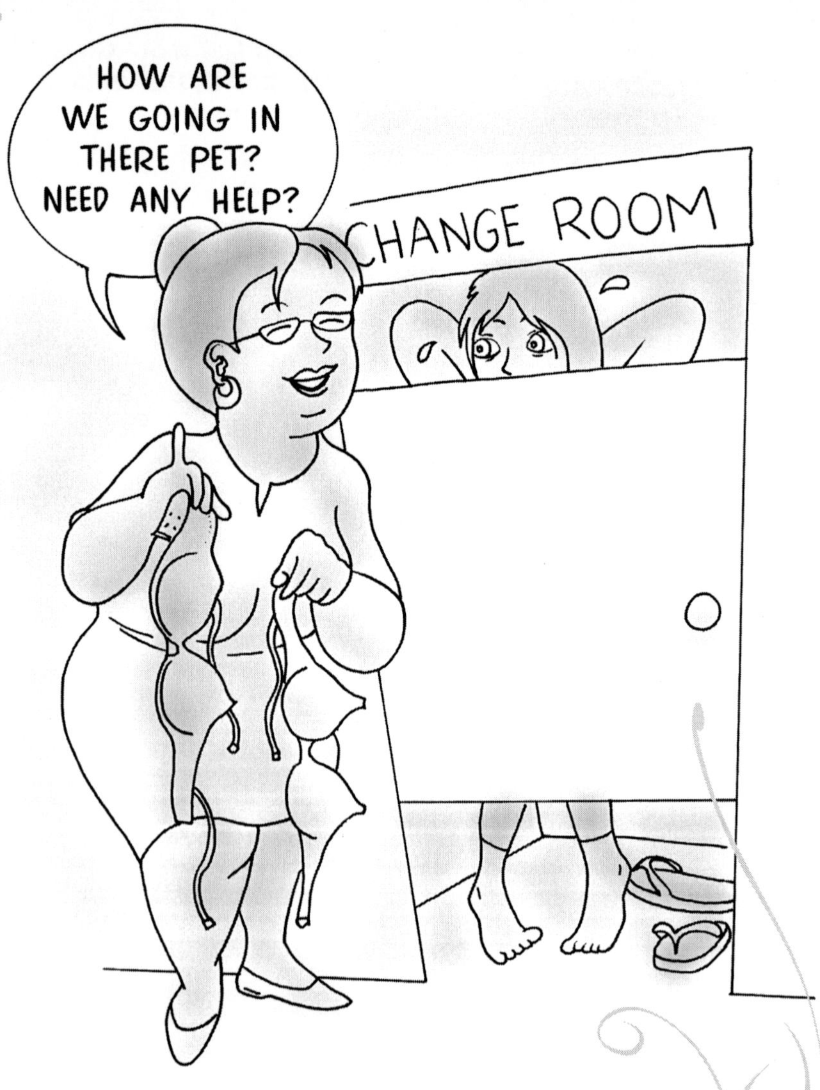
HOW ARE WE GOING IN THERE PET? NEED ANY HELP?
CHANGE ROOM

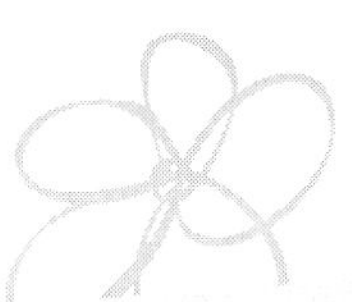

'My first bra fitting was a horrendous experience! I think I must have been about 13 years-old when my mum took me bra shopping at the local shopping centre. Unfortunately, the sales assistant was an older lady who had no sensitivity for a young girl whatsoever and kept flinging the change room curtain open to see how I was going. What's worse is, she kept bringing in increasingly smaller and smaller bras to try on. If the small bra sizes were not humiliating enough, the change room also faced the front entrance to the store which meant that each time the saleswoman flung open the curtain, anyone walking past could see me in my semi-naked state! Later that night, feeling like I had survived an initiation worse than anything else I could imagine, my mum noticed that I was wearing my new bra underneath my Pyjamas and announced in front of my dad that I didn't need to wear it to bed! I was so embarrassed! It was at that moment that I wished the ground would just swallow me up!'

'Back in the dim dark ages, when I was ready for my first bra, you had to be taken to get fitted! Imagine a 13 year-old, who is already embarrassed about everything, having to strip to the waist in a cubicle, and have an old lady fiddle with and measure your boobs! I will never forget it!! Added to that, the only suitable bra for "first timers" was all white, cotton, and pointy! What an easy time I gave my own daughters in comparison!'

'I was in Year 7 (first form) and had my lovely little pink bra that did up at the front. I remember being in English class when it somehow came undone! I whispered to my friend sitting next to me what had happened and she asked the teacher if I could go to the toilet. He agreed and I left with my arms crossed and gave my friend a look of warning that said, "Do not tell anyone!" I was out the door and walking away when I suddenly heard my entire class burst into laughter... I'll give you one guess why!'

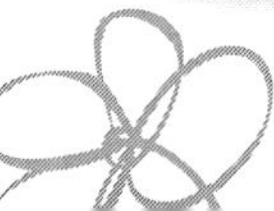

menstruation

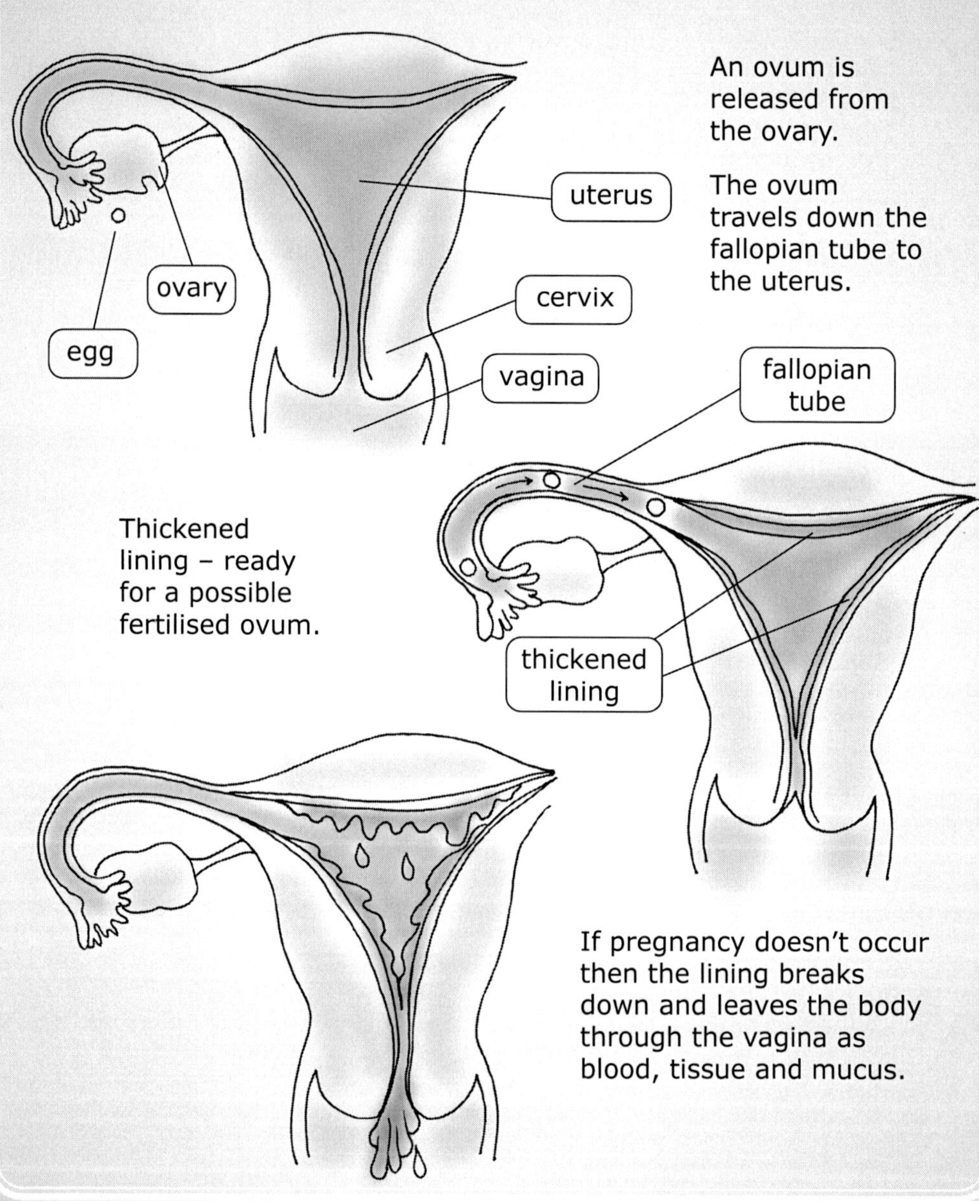

periods...

Menstruation

'Periods' are one of the most obvious signs to a girl that she has officially become a woman. Menstruation is the term used to describe the release of the lining of the uterus (womb) each month. It contains a small amount of blood flow which is actually made up of tissue, or cells, from the lining of the womb. You are not actually *bleeding* like when you cut yourself, rather you are discharging tissue and fluid that is not required because you are not having a baby.

What is menstruation?

Menstruation is the process by which eggs are released from a girl's ovary once per month. These egg cells are tiny, and can only be seen under a microscope. This entire process of the monthly cycle also involves the uterus (or womb) preparing for a possible pregnancy (which won't happen until you're much older!). The uterus prepares for a possible pregnancy by developing a lining made up of cells that will provide nutrients to a fertilised egg should this occur.

Menstruation is the process by which eggs are released from a girl's ovary once per month.

Unless a girl has been sexually active (had intercourse/sex) there is no way that an egg can be fertilised. This means that the uterus will not need the cells and mucous that it has prepared to nurture a fertilised egg. After a few days, the body realises that there is no fertilised egg, and begins to release the lining of the uterus, which is not needed anymore. This is the process of menstruation or 'having your period'.

>>>

The total amount of loss for each period is approximately 100mls (1/2 cup) and this loss occurs, on average, across 5–7 days each month, or every 28 days.

A girl can get her first period at any age; from 8 years-old right through to age 17. The average age, however, is usually between 11 and 14.

It is important to not worry about getting your period for the first time. It is a completely natural thing to happen and it is a sign that you are maturing into a gorgeous young woman, capable of having her own children one day!

A period is a completely natural thing to happen and it is a sign that you are maturing into a gorgeous young woman, capable of having her own children one day!

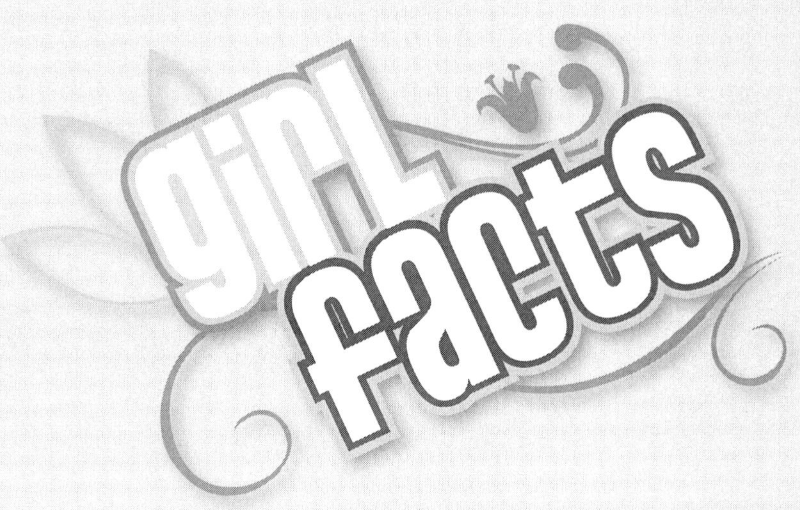

Girls are born with all the egg cells they will ever need, stored inside their two ovaries (pronounced ow-ver-ees). On average, each girl is born with thousands of eggs, each capable of being fertilised to produce a baby. Most of these eggs, however, are released and never used!

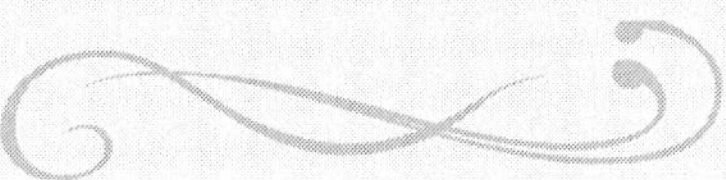

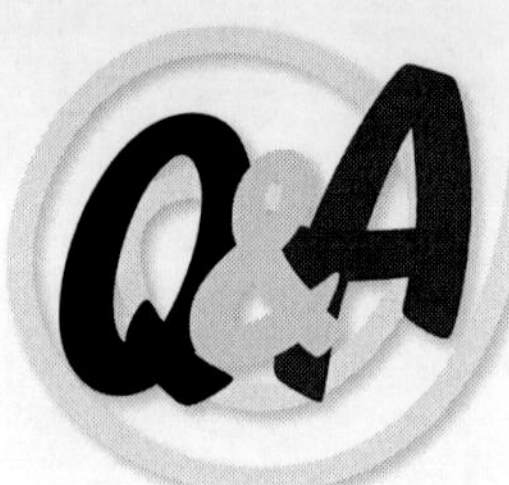

Why do we have to get our periods?

Most girls will eventually get their first period, and it is perfectly normal to feel a little anxious or worried about when and where this will first take place.

However, I would also like you to think of it as an exciting 'next step', as it means your reproductive system has woken up and your body is doing exactly what it has been created to do – prepare you for the chance to carry a baby one day if you choose.

If you feel nervous, or worried about the thought of getting your period, I encourage you to talk with a trusted female adult, or even one of your peers who has already begun this process.

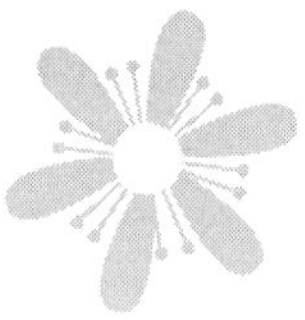

How often will I get my period?

In most cases, on average, girls will have a period roughly every 28 days. This counts from the first day you begin menstruating (not to be confused with 28 days after your period finishes – I made that mistake early on ☺)

Some girls experience their periods at longer intervals, such as every 35 days or longer. This is also perfectly normal, particularly in the first few months to a year of beginning as your body is adjusting and finding its own rhythm. If you have any concerns at all about the timing of your period, please chat to a trusted adult – mum, aunty, or teacher.

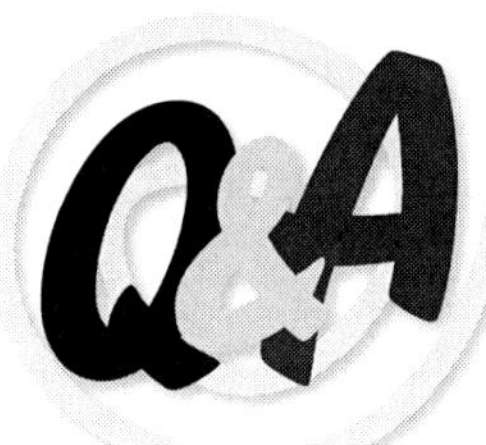

Is there something wrong with me? I still haven't got my period!

The first thing I'd like to say to you is, please try not to worry if you haven't begun getting your period. As each girl is at different stages of development during puberty, each will get their first period at any stage during this process. Whilst some girls will begin their puberty journey as early as late Primary School, others may be well into their High School years before it happens for them. I remember I was one of the later girls to get my period – closer to age 15, and I was not the last one out of my group of friends.

Just a side note on periods – it is very normal for your very first period to be a dark brownish colour, so be a little prepared for that. I had no idea, and it came as quite a shock to me the first time and I wasn't certain it was the arrival of my first period. After I chatted with mum, I was relieved to hear that yes, brownish blood was very normal.

...irregular periods?

As I mentioned earlier, it can take a few months or years for your period to get into a regular cycle. However, if you are concerned that they are months apart, or coming and going at odd times, it would be worth chatting to your trusted adult. They may suggest a visit to your doctor to see if there is something they can help to make your period more regular.

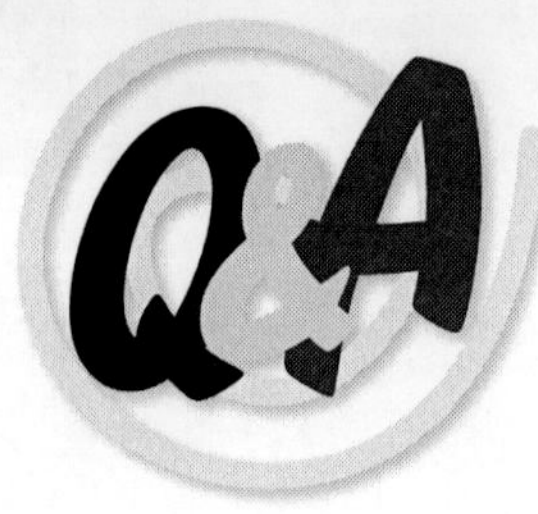

Is it normal to experience pain with my period?

When you have your period, you may experience mild discomfort in your stomach area. Some girls experience very difficult cramping, particularly during the first couple of days. This is not something to be concerned with, but it certainly can feel unpleasant. Cramping comes from the Uterus (which is a muscle) gently expanding and contracting as it releases its lining. Some girls don't feel much at all and go about life as normal. Others may need to take some pain medication, have warm baths, or use a heat pack on their stomach to help manage the cramps.

Helpful tips for pain with your period...

- *Take a warm bubble bath.*
- *Place a heat bag on your stomach and put your feet up.*
- *Sleep.*
- *Take some Paracetamol or consult your chemist if you experience extreme pain during these times.*
- *Walk or lightly exercise.*
- *Take a hot shower and let the water run on your back for a few minutes.*
- *Rest up and watch movies in bed or on the couch.*
- *Drink herbal tea.*

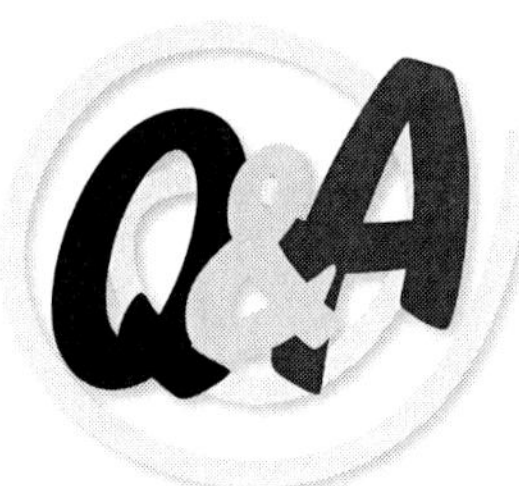

Why do my breasts hurt before I get my period?

Girls often experience breast swelling and/or tenderness in the week prior to getting their period. This is all a normal part of the cycle and occurs because our hormones are adjusting during our cycles. It's nothing to worry about, chat to a trusted adult if the pain becomes difficult to manage.

Should I use pads or tampons?

This is definitely a personal choice. Some girls use tampons from the very beginning of their periods, however most begin by using Sanitary pads. Sanitary pads are certainly a lot more user-friendly these days. The manufacturers have worked on great designs to make this part of your life just that bit easier.[1]

Many girls begin with pads in their early years, and may experiment with tampons later when they feel more comfortable. If you do intend to begin using tampons, it's a very good idea to read the instructions contained in the packet first. This is mainly because you do not want to injure yourself by trying to insert it incorrectly and also because there are certain guidelines that are important to follow.

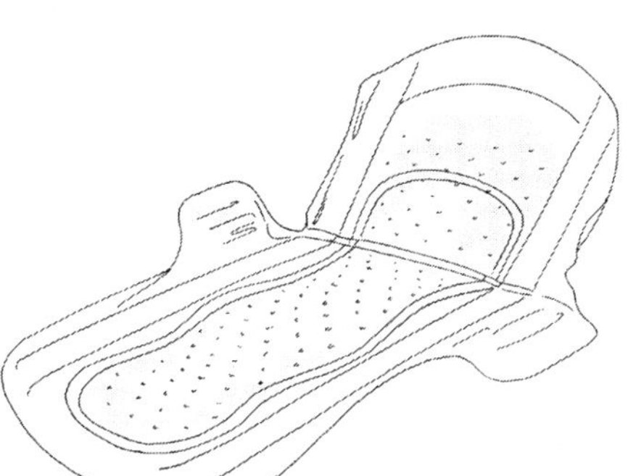

[1] You can now even purchase sanitary pads with wings! How wonderful is that!?! This is of course, to prevent leakage around your underwear.

Embracing comfort and helping the environment

With many girls wishing to focus on the effects of waste on our environment and sustainability, the development of period underwear has become a great option to using pads or tampons. Period underwear has been designed to use alongside, or in place of pads and tampons, offering a comfortable, leak-proof, and sustainable alternative.

Period underwear is created using advanced textile technology, featuring multiple layers that work together to provide protection against leaks and odors. The innermost layer is highly absorbent to keep you feeling dry. This layer is often followed by a waterproof barrier that prevents leaks from reaching your clothing. The outer layer is designed to be comfortable and stylish, resembling regular underwear while serving a special purpose.

- If you're **new to using period underwear**, it's important to choose the right size and absorbency level for your needs. Just like selecting any other period products, finding the right fit ensures optimal comfort and protection. Many brands offer a sizing guide on their websites to help you choose the right size based on your waist and hip measurements.
- **Wearing period underwear** is remarkably similar to wearing regular underwear. Simply put them on like you would with any other pair, making sure they fit snugly but comfortably. If you're using them as

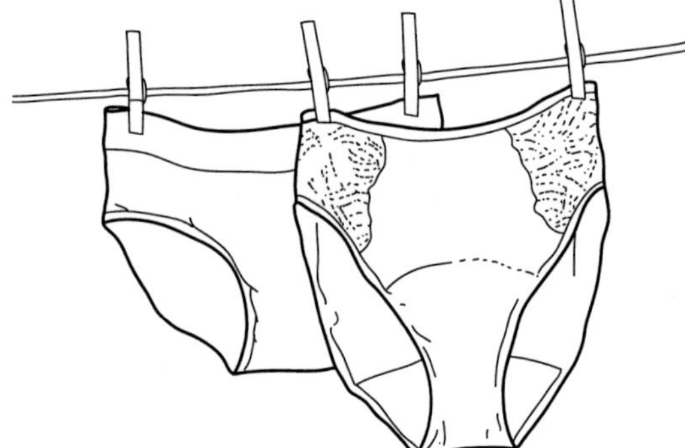

a replacement for traditional menstrual products, keep in mind that period underwear can typically hold the equivalent of 1 to 2 tampons' worth of fluid, depending on the brand and style.

- One of the key advantages of period underwear is the **comfort** it provides. Say goodbye to the discomfort of adhesive pads or the worry of tampon strings. With period underwear, you can move freely and confidently, knowing that you're protected against leaks.
- The **frequency of changing** period underwear depends on your flow. Just like with other period products, it's recommended to change them every 4-8 hours to ensure maximum freshness and leak protection. After removing them, rinse underwear in cold water to help prevent stains from setting. Then, simply toss them in the washing machine with your regular clothes.
- One of the most popular reasons to switch to period underwear is its **positive impact on the environment**. Disposable pads and tampons contribute to significant amounts of waste, whereas period underwear can last for years with proper care. By making the switch, you're reducing your carbon footprint and contributing to a more sustainable future.
- Period underwear is also an excellent option for **travel**. With no need to worry about packing a stash of disposable products or finding appropriate disposal methods, you can travel lighter and more confidently. The quick-drying properties of many period underwear brands make them convenient for on-the-go cleaning.

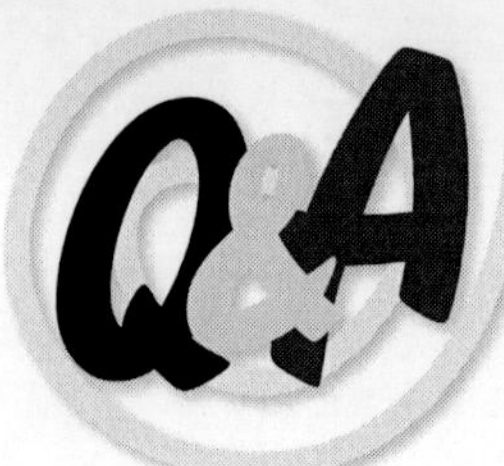

Why do you crave chocolate and ice cream when you have your period?

The sweet tooth cravings during your period are most likely your body's way of seeking comfort. Sugary sweets like chocolate and ice-cream can boost your Serotonin levels (those 'feel good' chemicals in your brain), making you feel happier, and more relaxed. It's like a little treat-yourself moment to make those period blues a bit more bearable. Just remember, it's totally normal, and indulging in some sweets can be a sweet escape during that time of the month.

Does it hurt when your hips change?

Some girls do experience some discomfort or mild pain when their hips change during puberty (a bit like growing pains). Puberty is a period of rapid growth and development, and it can bring about various physical changes, including widening of the hips. This widening is a natural part of your body's maturation process as it prepares for potential pregnancy and childbirth in the future.

It's important to note that while some discomfort can be normal during these changes, severe pain or persistent discomfort should be checked out by your doctor. Movement and regular exercise can also help.

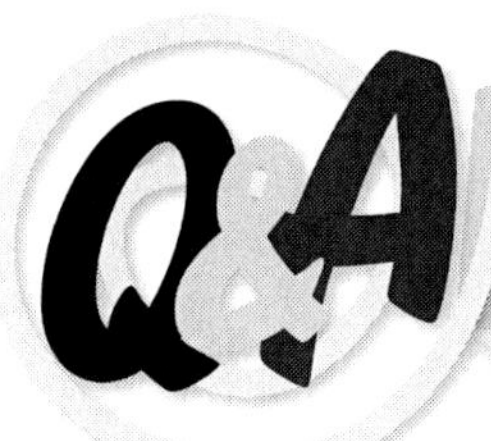

Do you still get your period when you are pregnant?

No, women do not get their period during pregnancy. This is because the lining of the uterus (that is usually expelled when a girl gets her period) is now needed to nourish the growing baby in the womb. During pregnancy, the body undergoes hormonal changes that prevent ovulation (the release of eggs from the ovaries) and the shedding of the lining of the uterus (womb.)

Is it weird if some parts of your body change before other parts?

It's completely normal for different parts of the body to change at different rates during puberty. It's a complex and individualised process that involves various hormonal, genetic, and environmental factors. As a result, the timing and order of physical changes can vary widely from person to person.

Does it mean I'm getting my period if I have pubic hair?

The development of pubic hair is one of the many changes that can occur during puberty, but having pubic hair alone is not a definitive sign that you are about to get your period. Pubic hair typically begins to develop in the early stages of puberty, which can start as early as 8-13 years old for girls.

Is it normal that around the dark part of my nipples there are little bumps?

Yes, the presence of small bumps around the dark part of the nipples (also known as areola), is perfectly normal. These bumps are called Montgomery glands, or Montgomery tubercles, and they are a natural part of the areola. The presence of Montgomery glands is not a cause for concern. They are a common and natural feature of the areola, and they serve an important function in maintaining the health and comfort of the nipple area. If you have any concerns about changes in your breasts or nipple area, it's always a good idea to consult a healthcare provider for reassurance and accurate information.

Is it normal to get rough armpits when you get armpit hair?

It's normal for the skin in the armpit area to become rough or textured when you start growing armpit hair. This change in texture is often due to a combination of factors, including the presence of hair follicles, oil glands, and potential friction from clothing. If you find that the rough texture is causing discomfort or irritation, there are steps you can take to care for your armpit skin:

- Moisturize: Applying a mild moisturizer or oil to the armpit area can help keep the skin hydrated and minimise roughness.
- Exfoliate: Gently exfoliating the area using a mild scrub or exfoliating cloth can help remove dead skin cells and improve the texture.
- Wear Breathable Fabrics: Choose clothing made from breathable materials to minimise friction and irritation.

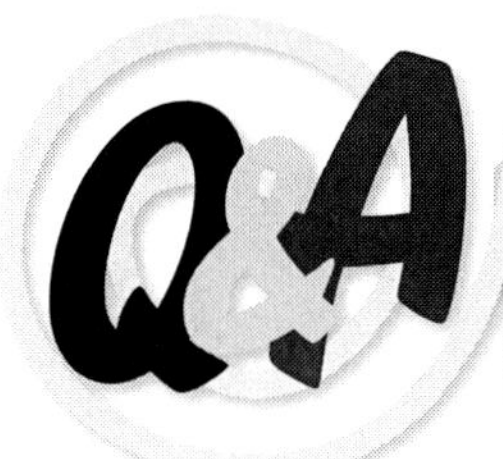

People tell me that you usually get your period at the same age your mum did, is this true?

It's a common belief that the age at which a girl gets their first period is often similar to when their mum or other female relatives began. While there can be a tendency for this to be true, it's not an absolute rule. The timing of getting your first period (menstruating) is influenced by a combination of genetic, hormonal, nutritional, and environmental factors, so there can be variations even among close relatives.

What if you don't get your period until you're older, like 18, and are too embarrassed to go to the doctor?

If you haven't started your period by the age of 18 and are feeling embarrassed or concerned about it, it's important to remember that you're not alone and there's no need to feel ashamed. While it's true that most girls begin their periods during their teenage years, the age at which menstruation begins can vary widely, and there's a broad range of what's considered normal.

If you are concerned that you haven't begun your period, it is worth sharing this with a trusted adult in your life. They may advise a visit to your doctor just to check your hormone levels and reassure you that all is okay. Try not to worry. ☺

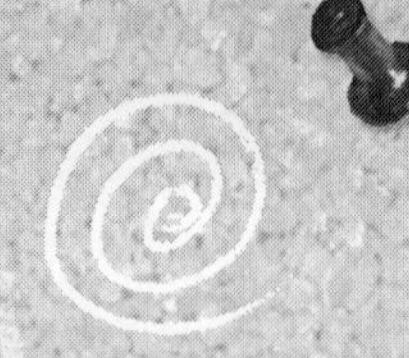

"In every aspect of our lives,
we are always
asking ourselves,
How am I of value?
What is my worth?
Yet I believe that
worthiness is
our birthright."
Oprah Winfrey
O' Magazne

"Be who you are and
say what you feel,
Because those who
mind don't matter,
And those that matter
don't mind."

Bernard M. Baruch

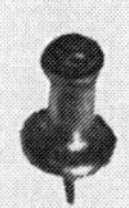

'Just be
yourself, there
is no one
better.'
Taylor Swift

"To be yourself in a world
that is constantly trying to make
you something else
is the greatest accomplishment."

Ralph Waldo Emerson

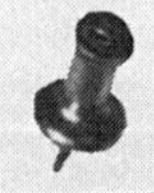

"You are you.
Now, isn't
that pleasant?"

Dr Seuss

"No one can make
you feel inferior
without your consent."

Eleanor Roosevelt

"Everybody wants
to be somebody;
nobody wants
to grow"

Johann von Goethe

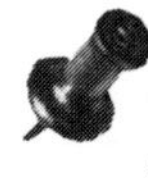

'Start treating yourself as if you're the most important asset you'll ever have. After all, aren't you?'
Anonymous

"Still round the corner there may wait, a new road or a secret gate."

J.R.R Tolkien

"Be yourself, everyone else is already taken."
Oscar Wilde

"A strong positive self image is the best possible preparation for success in life."

Joyce Brothers

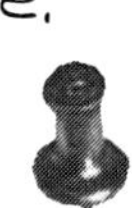

'Those who have a strong sense of love and belonging have the courage to be imperfect.'
Brene Brown

"Believe in your infinite potential. Your own limitations are those set upon yourself."

Roy T. Bemmet

'To shine your brightest light is to be who you truly are.'
Roy T Bennett

"Do what you can, with what you have, where you are."

Theodore Roosevelt

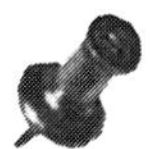

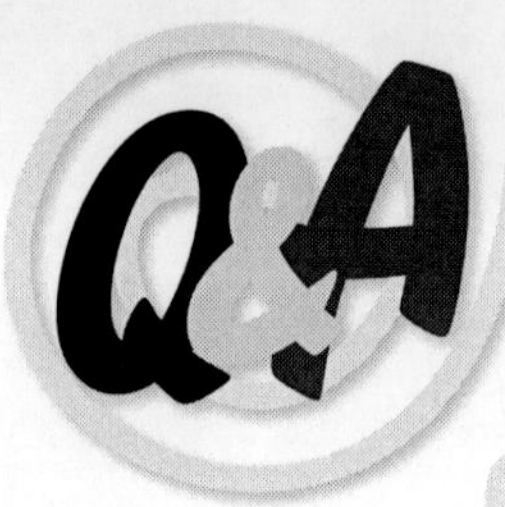

Change sanitary pads and tampons regularly

One of the most important things to remember is that feminine hygiene products — whether you are using pads or tampons — must be changed regularly! For hygiene reasons, this is of major importance. Pads that are not changed regularly can become smelly, also with tampons. They must be changed every 2-3 hours. Failing to change tampons regularly can lead to **Toxic Shock Syndrome** (caused by a common bacteria called Staphylococcus Aureus).

Common symptoms include:

- *High fever (over 38°)*
- *Vomiting*
- *Diarrhoea*
- *Sunburn-like rash*
- *Drop in blood pressure*
- *Muscle aches and pains*
- *Blood-shot eyes*
- *Confusion**

This information is not to scare you, but to educate you that people can develop this extreme and potentially life threatening illness caused by bacteria growing in the vagina.

If you ever experience any severe pain or discomfort during your period that doesn't feel normal, including headaches and temperatures, ***you must consult you doctor immediately.***

*Source: www.menstruation.com.au/periodpages/tss.html

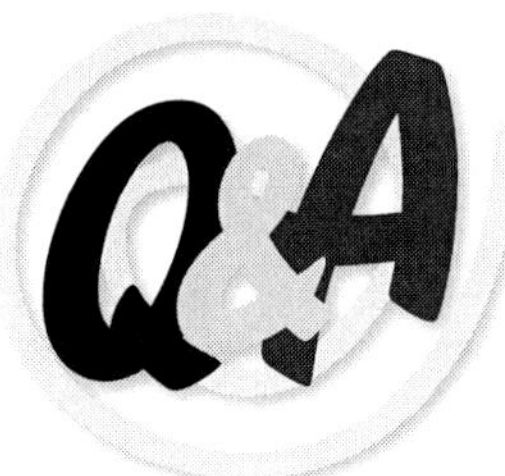

If I can't use a tampon, and pads are too big, what do I do?

Many girls don't feel comfortable at first using tampons, as they can take some getting use to. These days, however, pads have been produced that are very 'user friendly'. Many years ago pads were large, fat and *very uncomfortable*. The sanitary companies produce ultra thin pads that can barely be felt at all, once you are used to wearing them. They also stick securely to your underpants. You may also try using period underwear which are available at supermarkets or department stores, as well as online. (*See pages 58 & 59.*)

What if my period occurs at an inconvenient time?

If you were to ask most girls, they would tell you of an experience of getting their period at an 'inconvenient time'. Although many girls have a fairly accurate idea of when to expect their next period, sometimes, you may get it early or late. The good news here is that periods are perfectly normal and common among most teen girls and older women. If you're at school, let a friend know. Schools will usually have an 'emergency' supply of pads as will many of your girlfriends. Just remember, as awkward as it seems at the time, there is always a solution.

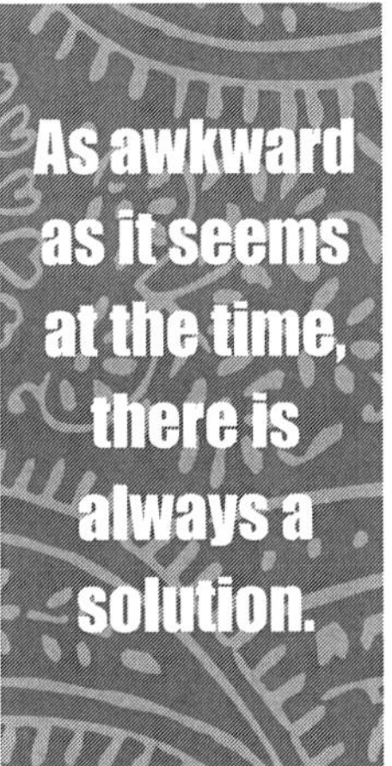

Take a deep breath, then ask for help. Folding up some toilet paper and placing it in your undies will buy you a little bit of time until you can reach some supplies! It's a great idea to carry spare supplies in your school bag or handbag.

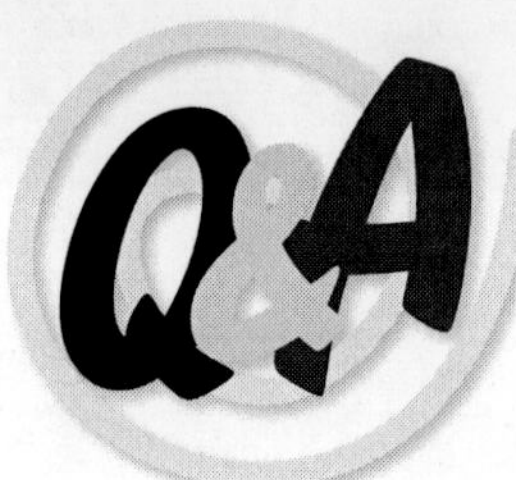

How do I know if I'm getting my period?

Some girls can feel a change in their emotions or moods just before their period starts. Some girls also experience slight tenderness in their breasts, and others feel a bit bloated around their tummy area. Other girls experience no warning signs at all. Just remember, whatever your experience, it's normal for you!

How do you use a tampon?

Tampons are inserted into the vagina to absorb the flow during menstruation. It is usually inserted using a clean finger, however some companies provide applicators that can help with this process. Using tampons for the first time can be quite tricky. You need to be relaxed and certainly don't try it for the first time if you are in a rush and feeling stressed.

How can you prevent leaking?

The best way to prevent leaking during your period is to remember to change your pad or tampon regularly; eg: every 2-3 hours. You can also use pads that have specially designed wings on either side that fold over the undersides of your undies.

Am I too young to wear a g string?

A g string is basically a pair of underwear that has a 'string-like' back to it. If a teen girls chooses to wear a g string, that is her personal choice and an issue of comfort. There are no medical reasons why you cannot wear a g string. When you have your period though, normal underwear is better if you use pads.

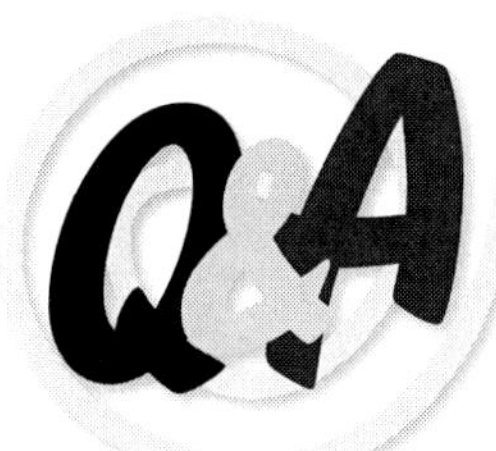

What happens if I go swimming with my period?

If you are wearing a tampon,
it is perfectly fine to swim whilst you have your period. If you are using pads, it's best to give swimming a miss as **they can never be used for swimming**. Some girls say that when you swim, you won't discharge any blood. That is not usually the case and it is certainly not worth the risk of embarrassment. If by chance you are at a swimming carnival at school or on camp and you suddenly get your period, politely ask to speak to one of the female teachers. They will most certainly understand and should excuse you from participating in swimming. You can also buy specific period underwear as bathers.

keep yourself clean!

This should be quite obvious, however, some girls need to be reminded that you must bath or shower daily when you have your period! Some girls who experience a particularly heavy flow may even need to shower twice a day. Whatever is required, make sure you keep yourself clean and comfortable. Sometimes you may experience a strong unpleasant odour with your period. This could be caused by blood left on your pubic hair from the pad. Once air gets to it, you may experience a bad odour. So it's important to clean yourself well and shower regularly.

If you are on school camp and cannot get to a shower as often as you'd like, dampen down a face washer with warm water and clean yourself thoroughly. Even though this might sound like a pain, it is worth saving the embarrassment of having other people thinking you smell!

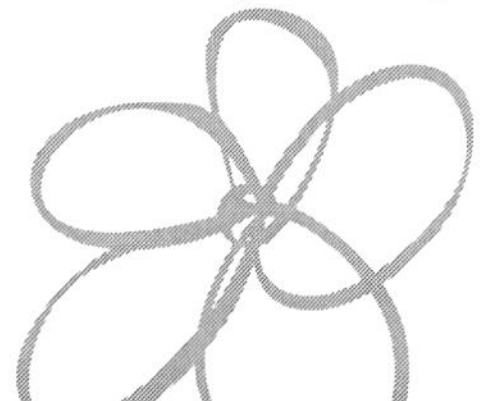

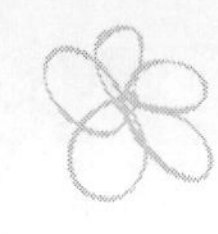

How long should my period last?

In terms of your life, unfortunately we're talking at least about 35 years ☺. That's a bit of a bummer! In terms of every month, the simple answer is 3–7 days, though once again, this may vary. If it lasts any longer than 10 days, you should check in with your doctor. Most girls fall around the 5–6 day category, however it is not uncommon for menstruation to last up to 7 days.

Be prepared!

Always be prepared for the possibility of getting your period. This is not to make you feel scared at all, but it's a good idea to have something in the bottom of your school bag from the age of 10 or 11, just in case. Unfortunately, your period doesn't often come with a warning. You may have no idea at all that you are getting it. Try organising a small funky looking pencil case or cute purse. Pop in a couple of pads so that you are prepared just in case!

If you are going on camp or will be away from home for a few days, take your emergency pack with you.

If you are going on camp or will be away from home for a few days, take your emergency pack with you. Many companies will send you a sample pack for free. You may even receive a pack at school during your personal development studies.

period calendar

Can you know when your period will happen?

Generally speaking, once your menstrual cycle is settled, you should expect to get your period every 28 days. This can vary, and it can take some time to settle down at the beginning of your periods. In the beginning, you may only get your period every six weeks or longer. The average however is 28 days so we will use this for our example below.

You can work out when your period is due next by calculating from day 1 of your period. Count from day 1 and when you get to day 28, this is when you *should* get your next period. Using a calendar or a diary is the best way of calculating this and reminding yourself to be prepared.

Nowadays you can also download period apps that are a brilliant tool to help you keep track of your period.

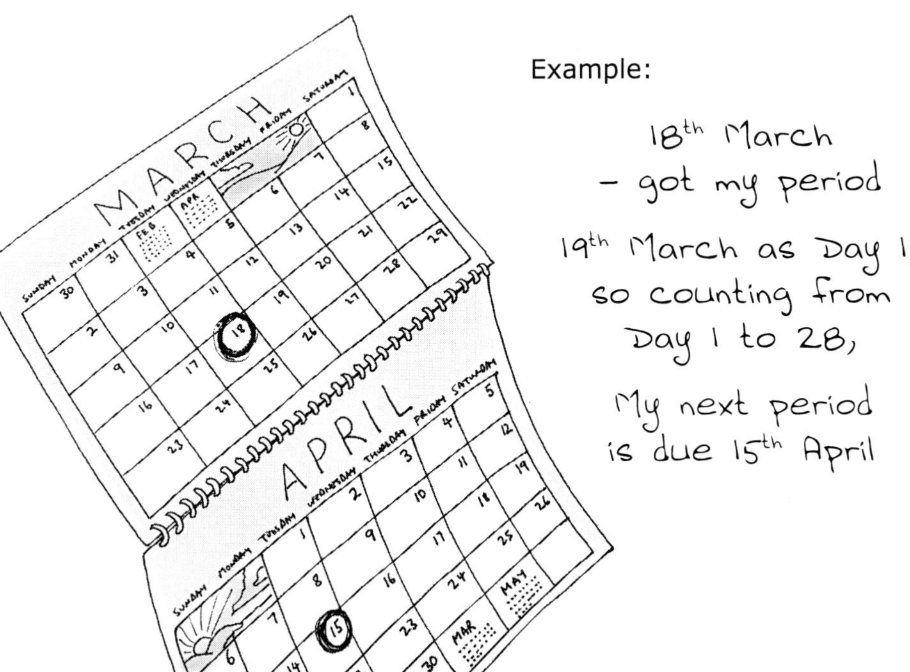

Example:

18th March – got my period

19th March as Day 1, so counting from Day 1 to 28,

My next period is due 15th April

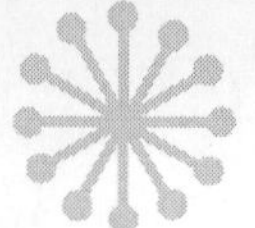

girl's experiences...

A collection of memories and anecdotes from girls and women who've survived their period experiences...

'When I first got my period it was really hard because my mum never had her period due to a medical condition. She never said a word about it to prepare me and being the eldest, I was not prepared at all. I felt very alone! I got my period around age 17. I remember that it felt quite late, and boy, ***was it a shock to the system!*** *I was totally unsure of how to deal with getting my first period. It was embarrassing for me to have to try and deal with all these changes going on with my body, especially practically. What methods were best? What practical techniques? What should I use?*

I was so embarrassed once when I was caught out by my brothers with undies soaking in the bathroom sink, where I accidentally left them soaking when I was in the shower. The times that girls have reason for toilet stops for changing pads is a very alone time, especially being a girl in between two boys in the family. ***I guess all girls struggle to some degree****, but being sports crazy made it all the more difficult for me.*

Getting your period certainly does affect your body and your energy levels can be very much hindered depending on the type of person you are. For me, the difficulty was the whole process of carrying replacements and disposing of items after use. There are not always the correct bins supplied, especially at home with a family and all boys around. How embarrassing!'

'I remember during my Year 10 Cross Country run, about halfway through, I discovered that I had my period and it was really heavy! In fact, it was fairly obvious considering I was wearing bloomers and a short PE skirt. I had absolutely NO supplies with me at school and had to make my way to a friend's locker so I could go to the toilet. Of course, the male teachers who were supervising the race saw me and immediately thought I was cheating! I had to explain to about three teachers why I couldn't finish the race. Being the incredibly shy teenager that I was, I was mortified!'

'It can actually be quite stressful for a young girl getting her period. There is so much that is so new that they need to learn.'

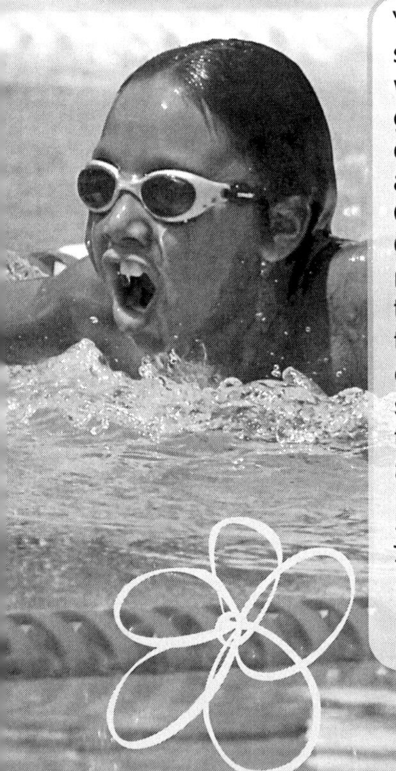

'I remember that my period was always so unreliable so I never knew when I was going to get it. I was a sports-mad girl which didn't help. I remember one day when I got my period, just as I was about to race in our Swimming Sports Carnival at school. Because I was Sports Girl of the Year for the previous four years running, there was absolutely no way that I could miss out! Every race counted towards the trophy! Normally, if a girl got her period on sports day they would simply take the day off. But not me. I had to try someone's rescue solution — ***the tampon***! I had never tried one before but I just had to race! Some things are just more important hey? I had no idea that girls could only swim with a tampon. Luckily my friend came to the rescue and I went on to win the race!'

'I remember that I got my period in about Year 9, which felt quite late but was pretty normal for my age. One day, I got my period at school when I was totally unprepared for it. I called out to one of my friends in the next toilet cubicle. She went down to the office to get something for me to use. Well I nearly fell off the toilet seat when she passed under the toilet door what could best be described as some sort of pillow that you'd use for a doll! I nearly died! We were both laughing but I was so embarrassed. I had to use it because I had no alternative at the time. As I walked out of the toilets I felt as if I had a giant nappy in between my legs and I'm sure I walked with a waddle! This incident has left such an impression on me that now, as a Middle School teacher, I have a special 'Secret Girl's Box' in my storeroom that all girls can use — just to save the embarrassment of having to use anything that the office ladies can find.'

'I got my period just after turning 12. I still remember the moment as it was my sister's birthday. I really thought my life was over! (being the Drama Queen that I was). I remember going to my room and crying, unsure of what to do. Perhaps mum hadn't spoken to me enough about it. I felt so alone as I was the first in my class to get it and I was only in grade six!'

'I got my period on December 14, 1997. I was 14. I looked in my undies for the entire year before waiting..... just waiting for what my mum said would be the first sign that I was now officially a woman. Finally, I became one! I phoned my dad and he was so proud!'

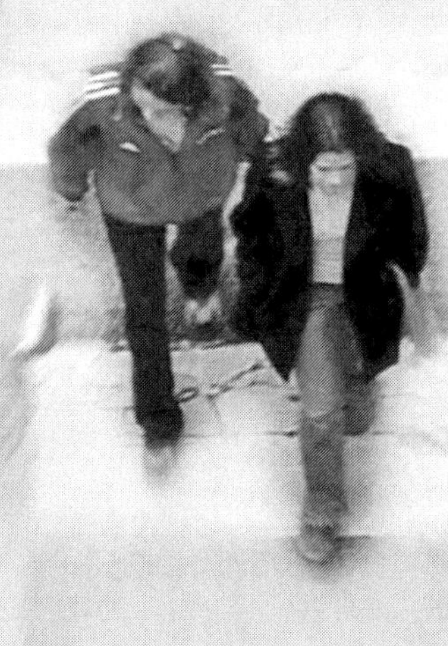

'Getting my period for the first time couldn't have been worse! I remember I was on guide camp holiday. Our leader was the heartless type. It was all so embarrassing to come to terms with this new stage of your development and not having any privacy. I was 13½ years-old and remember to this day being horrified in a Portaloo whilst on camp. I experienced cramps and shock at the reality of it all. The worst thing was having no one to talk to about it. I felt alienated and deeply embarrassed. I vowed that if I ever had a daughter, this would become a day to celebrate together. When my daughter did get her period, we had a great day out shopping, with some pampering to make it a memorable day!'

'My most embarrassing moment with my period was one time when I went to the movies with my mum. We went to watch "Maid in Manhattan". Well, the movie ended and I proceeded to stand up and exit the cinema. But alas, my period had soaked through everything — my knickers, my pants, everything!! and not just lightly... I'm talking torrential flood!! I must have been thoroughly engrossed in the movie because I hadn't felt a thing. I totally freaked out! I was trying to avoid people noticing me at all costs. We tied my denim jacket around my waist to disguise the situation and proceeded to waddle uncomfortably back to the car where I sat on a crackly plastic bag for the entire car trip home.

Lesson learnt: Always take a toilet break at the movies!'

'My Grandmother got her period when she was 10 years-old! Nobody had told her anything about periods and she immediately thought she was dying. I often think about how awful that must have been for her.'

'I first got my period at school and I will never forget it! I knew all about periods (I was the last one in my class to get it) but I was totally unprepared for it happening at school. I had no pads or tampons with me and was too embarrassed to ask a friend or teacher for help so I scrunched up some toilet paper in my undies. It was that shiny, awful, hard toilet paper that we used to have in our school and it was very uncomfortable!'

'In my husband Greg's family, things such as periods were never talked about, well at least to the males in the house. Greg's mum had a code word that she used whenever his sister had her period. She would say, "Mandy can't go swimming today because she has a sore leg". Now Greg and I often refer to periods in our household as "having a sore leg!".'

'One day, as I was watching a movie, I noticed a wetness in my shorts. I paused the DVD and went to my room because I thought I'd either wet myself or something else was seriously wrong with me. When I looked in my underpants, I saw that they were literally covered in blood. I went to mum and told her I thought I had my period. She confirmed this to be true. Wearing a pad was uncomfortable at first but I've gotten use to it. Note to self: NEVER wear white shorts at aged 14 if you haven't got your period yet!'

'I remember at age 13, staying at my friend's house for a sleepover, when my period came totally unannounced! I wasn't prepared at all! I didn't know what to do. I barely knew my friend's mum to say anything to her and I certainly didn't want to tell my friend as I felt too embarrassed that I didn't come prepared. Sooooo, I rolled up some pieces of toilet paper until I thought it looked like a tampon and proceeded to use that. Unfortunately, the toilet paper was a lovely shade of apricot so it didn't really look like a tampon at all. Anyhow, once I was sorted, off to the park we went on our bikes to meet up with our boyfriends. Naturally, nature took it's course and my period leaked everywhere, all through my denim jeans onto the yellow bike seat. It turns out that toilet paper isn't half as absorbent as tampons (I wish somebody had told me that earlier!). To my horror, my boyfriend Johnny noticed the blood on the bike seat. When he said, "What's that on your bike seat?" I replied, "Oh, I just cut my leg". He simply shrugged and carried on doing jumps on his bike. Isn't it fantastic that 13 year-old males really don't have much of a clue about what's going on with girls and will pretty much believe anything you tell them? Poor Johnny really was clueless and consequently he was dumped a week later!'

'I remember when I got my period I was going to have a shower and I needed to go to the toilet. When I got there, I had blood in my pants, so I went in to see mum but she was on the phone. So I went to tell my sister and she gave me a pad to put on after I had a shower. It was so uncomfortable and very wet.'

PUBIC hair

Pubic hair is one of the other unexciting things we have to cope with as we begin developing our adult bodies. It can be quite daunting to one day find bits of scraggly hair poking out from under your arm or in your pubic region. Let's be perfectly honest here and say that it's not the most exciting thing for us to cope with as girls. We usually want to shave the hair off from under our arms and on our legs as soon as we can. As with periods, pubic hair can develop from 9 years of age right through to 15 or 16 years; all is within the realm of normality! Just remember that once you begin shaving under your arms, the hair will begin to grow back thick and fast so you will find yourself doing this regularly for the next 70 years or so, depending on what you decide.

I also want you to know that, despite what society norms may be and the images you are bombarded with on social media, you DON'T HAVE TO remove any pubic hair. It's a personal choice. Be YOU!

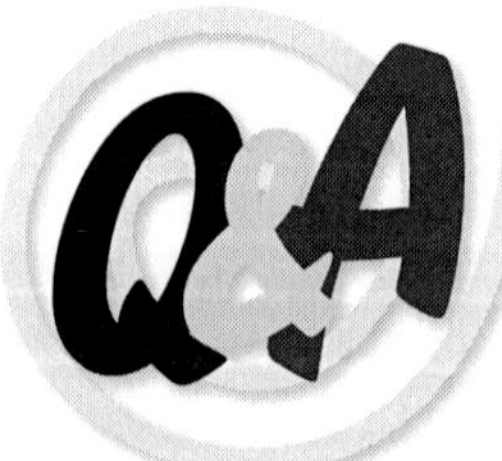

Why do we get pubic hair?

When asked this very question by a group of 12 year-old girls once, my immediate response was 'for cushioning effects', to which another teacher laughed and replied, 'I don't think that's right!'. We had a good laugh about it at the time, but it was a pretty good question. The main reason is that pubic hair is a temperature regulator. When we sweat in these areas, the hairs help to keep the body's temperature at normal levels.

three//

The inside story

Babies, pregnancy and birth

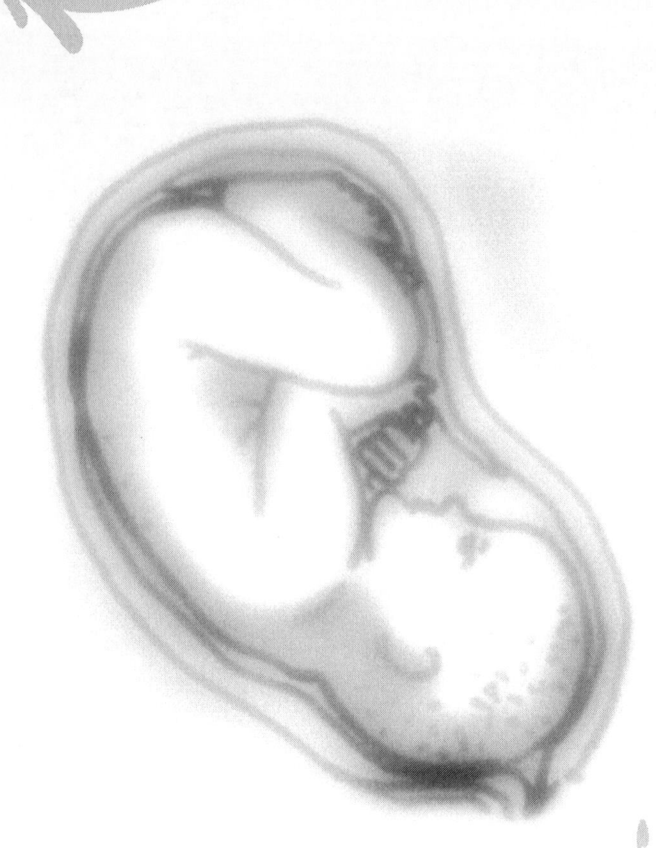

The miracle of creating and

bringing a baby into the world

is a truly wonderful

blessing

fertilisation of a baby

The miracle of creating and bringing a baby into the world is a truly wonderful blessing.

It is something to be celebrated as it is such a miracle. This chapter explains some of the more physical parts of conceiving (making) a baby and how it grows inside its mother in preparation for beginning an amazing life outside of the womb.

Conception

Conception of a baby involves the union between a male and a female. This is what is most commonly known as *sex* or ***sexual intercourse***. During sexual intercourse, the man's penis enters the woman's vagina. The couple move in and out in a way that feels pleasurable to them both. During this process, an ejaculation is released from the man's penis into the woman's vagina. This contains semen, which is a whitish liquid containing sperm. Sperm are the tiny, microscopic cells that are needed to meet with a female's egg in order to make a baby.

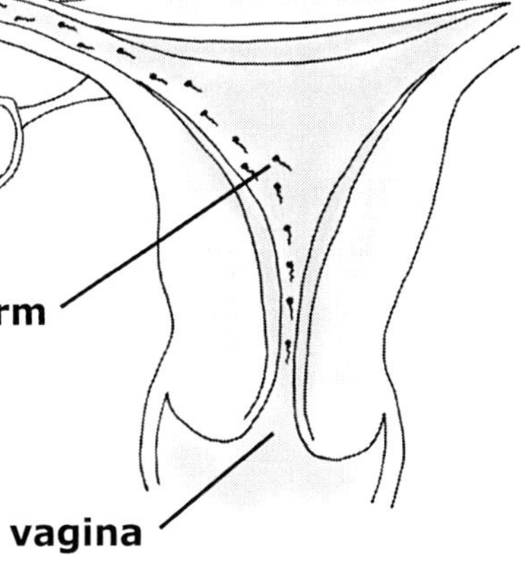

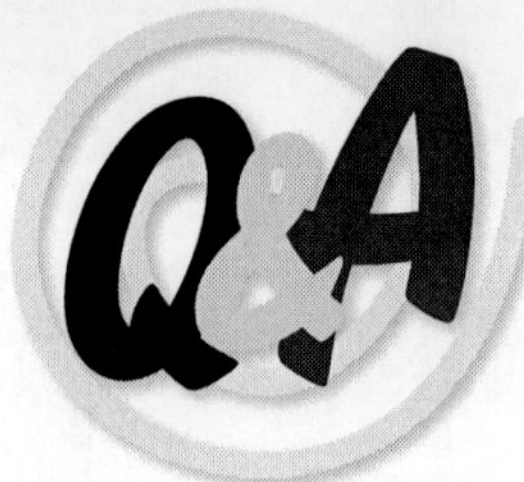

Can a woman get pregnant each time she has sexual intercourse?

No, a woman will not become pregnant each time she has intercourse. This is because there are only certain times during each month that a woman is ovulating.

Ovulation is the time each month when an egg is released from one of the female's **ovaries** and enters the **fallopian tube**. The egg cell will only remain in the fallopian tube for a few days. If it is fertilised by a sperm cell during this time, then the fertilised egg will move down into the woman's uterus (more commonly known as the womb), where it will hopefully continue developing for the next nine months into a healthy baby.

How many sperm cells are needed to fertilise the woman's egg?

Only one! Now that is pretty incredible considering that there are millions of tiny sperm cells in each ejaculation of semen. But the very moment that one sperm cell fertilises a woman's egg, a protective barrier is formed around the egg immediately, and no other sperm cells can penetrate it.

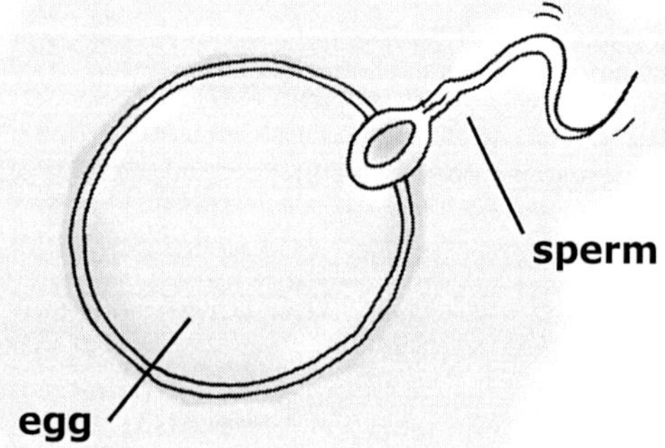

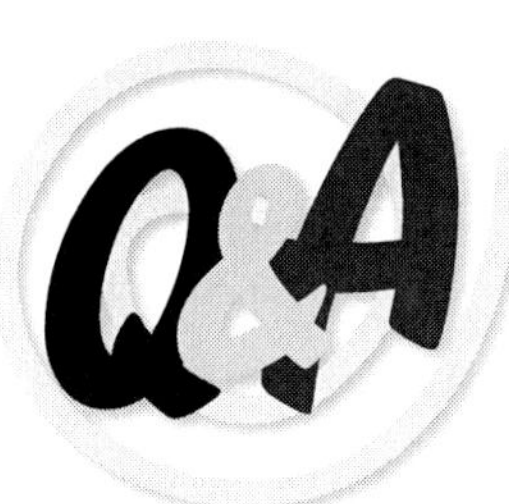

Why have sex even if husbands and wives don't want to get pregnant?

Sexual intercourse is also a very pleasurable way for a committed couple to express their deep love for each other. Making babies is just a part of having a healthy, sexual relationship.

What happens if a woman does not want to get pregnant?

If a woman is not ready to have a baby, there are certain things that can be done to prevent the sperm reaching the egg. Sometimes a man will wear a condom on his erect penis, which will prevent the fluid entering the vagina. A woman can also use a variety of medications and other medical options. This prevents ovulation during the monthly cycle. Even though she will still get her period each month, she will not release an egg from her ovary.

Why do girls have two ovaries?

When girls are born, both ovaries contain all the reproductive egg cells she will ever need to fertilise a baby. Each month, the ovaries take turns releasing an egg for possible fertilisation. If the left ovary releases an egg on one month, the next month, the right ovary will usually release an egg and so on.

Pregnancy

Having a baby is usually a happy and very exciting time for all concerned. Pregnancies last for 40 weeks, or nine months from the day of conception. During that time, a woman's body goes through many changes as it accommodates a fast growing baby.

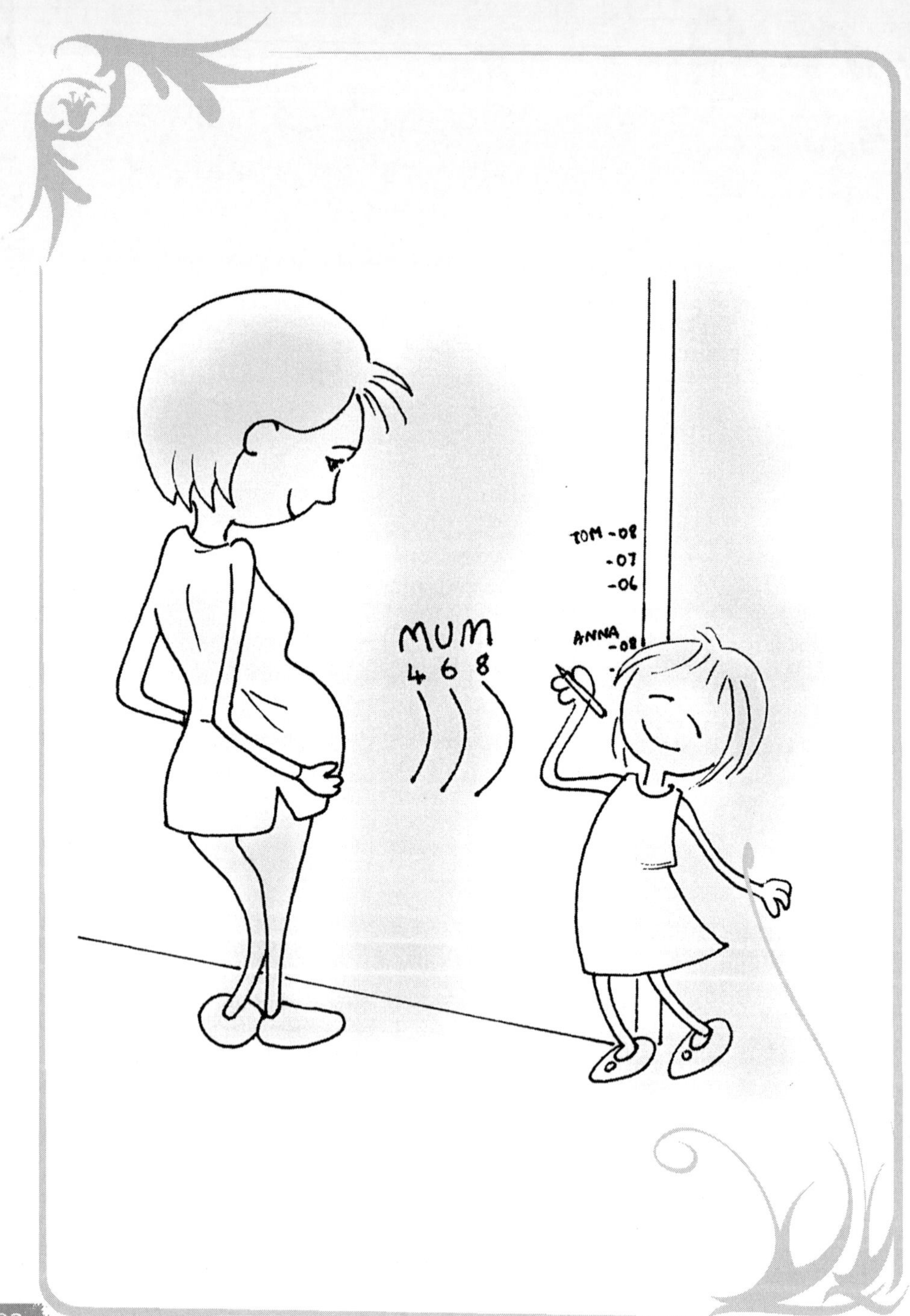
TOM -08
-07
-06
MUM
4 6 8
ANNA
-08

how does a woman know she is pregnant?

Sometimes a woman will know fairly quickly that she is expecting a baby because she misses her regular period. Because a baby has been fertilised and is now growing in the uterus (womb), the lining does not need to be expelled, so her period will not come. This is when most women will take a home pregnancy test or go to a doctor to have a test to confirm a baby has been conceived.

Some other symptoms that a woman may experience during her pregnancy include:

- Increase in appetite.
- Morning sickness, feeling nauseous.
- Tenderness in breasts.
- Increased tiredness.

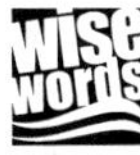

Before I shaped you
in the womb,
I knew all about you.
Before you saw the
light of day,
I had holy plans
for you.

Jeremiah 1:5
(The Message)

A woman will know fairly quickly that she is expecting a baby because she misses her regular period.

the Stages of pregnancy

6 weeks, *budding forth*

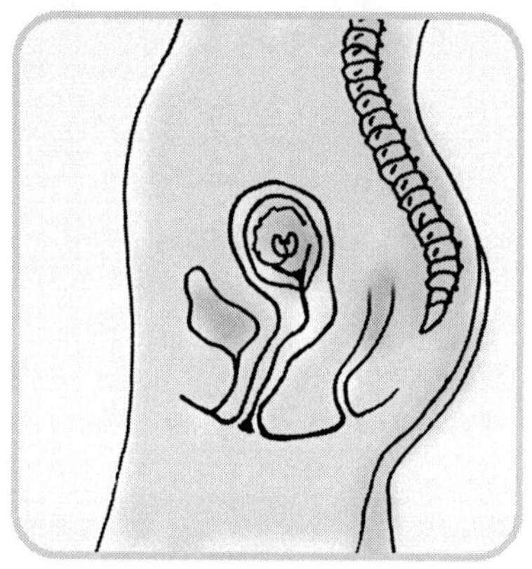

At six weeks, the fertilised baby is known as an **embryo**. It is less than 1.5cm in length and will be the shape of a jelly bean or large peanut. The buds which will form the arms and legs are just beginning to show.

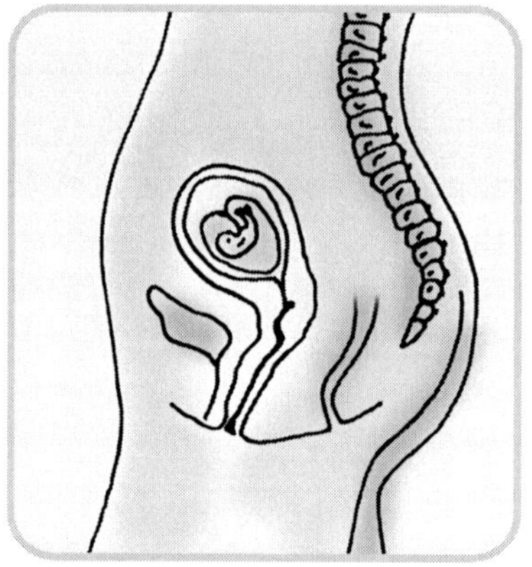

12 weeks, *there's a baby in there*

The baby is now known as a **foetus** at 12 weeks gestation. It is approximately 9cm in length and weighs about 140 grams. It now is beginning to look a bit more like a baby!

20 weeks, *first peek*

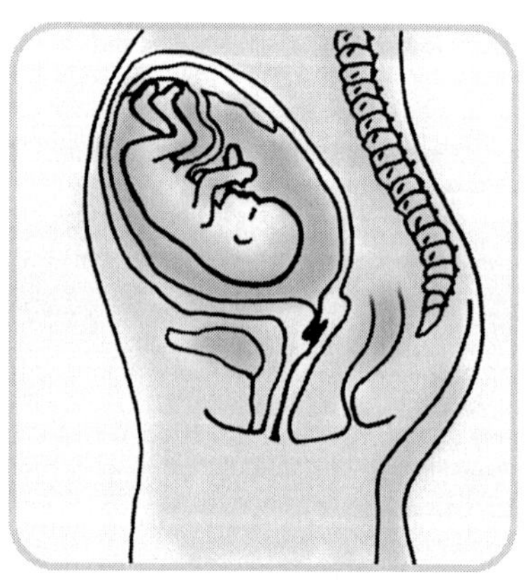

This is now the official halfway mark of the pregnancy. Most women can begin to feel the baby moving inside her by now. The foetus is now about 25cm long and weighs around 300 grams. Many women have an ultra sound scan at this stage of the pregnancy.

This involves a scan at a clinic or hospital in which an image is displayed of the baby on a monitor. It is possible to tell whether the baby is going to be a girl or a boy at this stage.

32 weeks, *moving out of home soon*

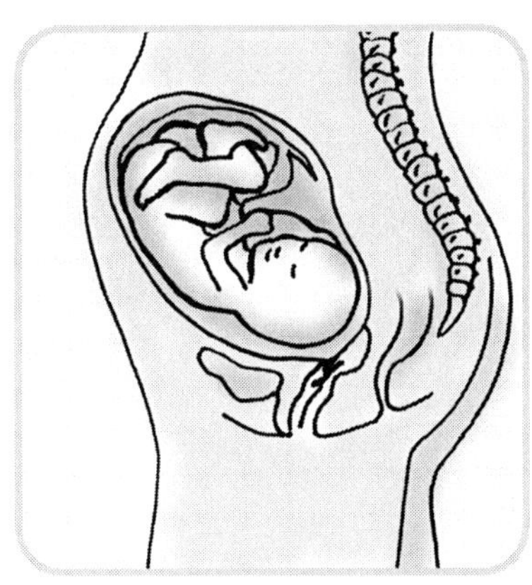

The baby is fully formed at this stage of the pregnancy, although the lungs would still not be strong enough to work well if born. If born, the baby might possibly survive if receiving expert care from a hospital. The baby is now approximately 43cm in length from head to toe and would weigh around 1800 grams. From this stage, the baby will be quite active in a mother's womb. For the last 4 weeks of a mother's pregnancy, the baby will mostly just gain weight and prepare for its big entry!

40 weeks, *hello world!*

The baby is now full term and ready to begin life in the world. Quite often, the mother will feel very tired and may also experience Braxton Hicks (practice contractions).

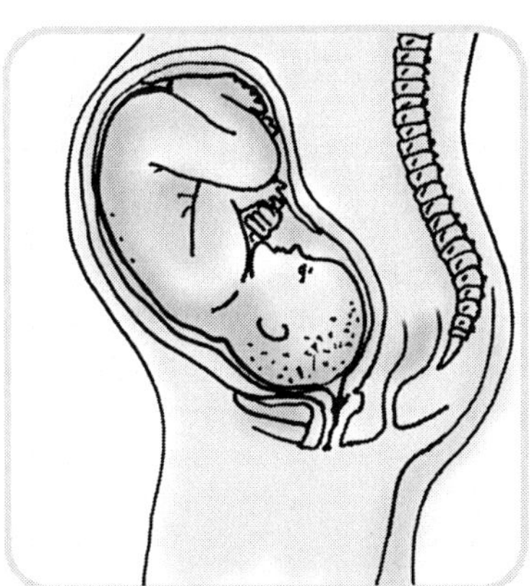

The contractions are what will be needed to bring the baby through the woman's birth canal (vagina) and into the world. The average full term baby will weigh around 3500 grams and measure 50cm long, however this can vary quite a lot with each pregnancy.

Childbirth

Labour begins when the baby is around 40 weeks gestation (this means it has 40 weeks of growing in the womb). Sometimes, a woman will begin to experience period-like cramps at the beginning, whilst some will feel their water break, which is the amniotic fluid that surrounds the baby in the womb. Once this breaks, the fluid can leak out through the vagina, and this is a sure sign that the baby is getting ready to make its way out. The process of labour can be divided into three sections:

First stage of labour

The first stage of labour is often the longest, but not always.

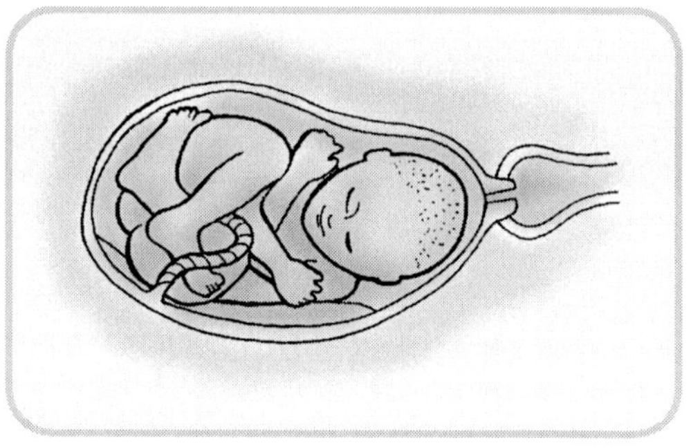

During the first stage of labour, contractions cause the cervix to open or dilate. The cervix is located at the top of the vagina, at the opening of the womb. This is usually the longest stage of labour because the cervix must open (dilate) to 10cm so that the baby's head is able to pass through. Although some women are able to walk around during the first stage, it can become quite painful as the contractions become stronger and more frequent. Once the cervix has stretched to 10cm, the baby can then be delivered.

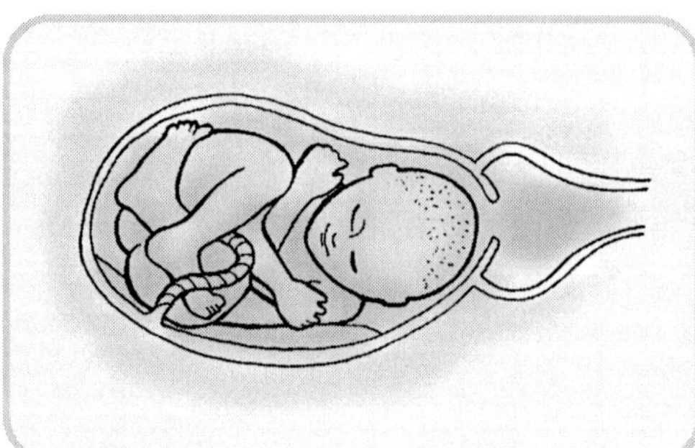

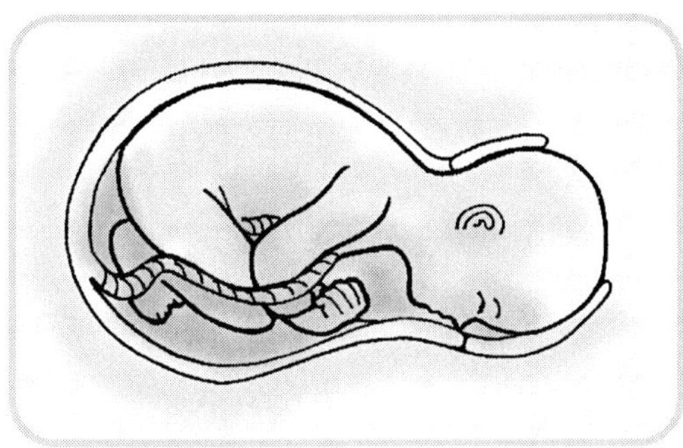

Second stage of labour

During the second stage of labour, the baby is delivered.

During each contraction, the baby is moved by the body's muscles down through the birth passage (the vagina). Once the baby's head reaches the entrance to the vagina (known as crowning) the mother can then push the baby out head first. This is quite often painful but also a truly incredible and wonderful experience.

Third stage of labour

During the third stage of labour, once the baby has been safely delivered, the **placenta** needs to be delivered. The placenta is the thick membrane-like sack that has been housing the baby for the past 40 weeks and providing nutrients to the growing baby. It is essential that this is removed through another series of contractions immediately after the birth. This is why the placenta is also known as the **afterbirth**.

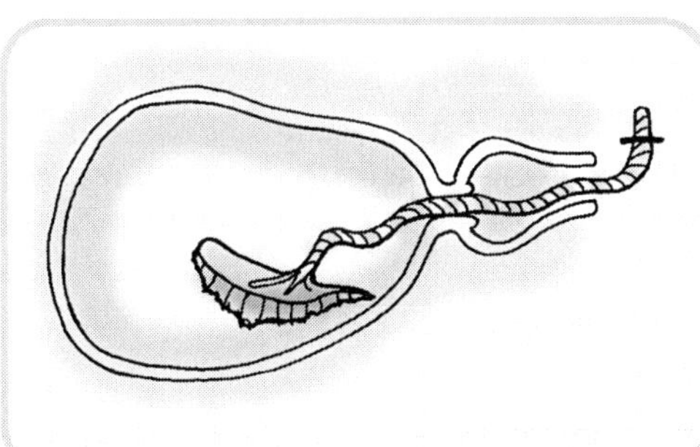

Why are babies covered in blood and white stuff?

Because the placenta contains blood, the baby will often have some of this on their body. The white coating on the baby's skin is called **vernix**. This is a barrier-like substance that covers the baby's skin during pregnancy to prevent it getting all wrinkly. In fact, they swim in liquid inside the placenta for the entire 40 weeks. Some babies are covered in a lot of vernix when they are born, whilst some don't have much at all.

How painful is childbirth? it sounds scary!

Labour can be a painful experience, however the experience of pain is different for each woman. Some women use a variety of relaxation techniques during labour, such as having a bath, massage and listening to relaxation music. Other types of pain relief are available if a woman requires it, such as gas, or painkillers. There is also the availability of an Epidural Injection, where a spinal block is inserted into the lower spine that causes numbness from the waist down. There is nothing to fear with childbirth, as there are many types of pain relief available.

What is a Caesarean?

Sometimes for a variety of reasons a vaginal delivery is not possible. In this case a mother will be under anaesthetic while a surgeon delivers the baby through an incision (cut) into the lower abdomen. This is called a caesarean or caesarean section.

four //

caring for your health

Tips for Staying Healthy!

- *Shower daily*
- *Use a good anti-perspirant deodorant*
- *Wash/and clean your face daily*
- *Get lots of sleep (aim for 8–10 hours)*
- *Drink plenty of water (8 glasses per day is what you should aim for!)*
- *Brush and floss your teeth twice daily!*

staying healthy

It's important to keep healthy during puberty and as you grow into a young woman. As you enter puberty, you'll notice an increase in your sweat — particularly your underarms. As you begin menstruation, it is even more important to shower daily.

If you find that you sweat a lot, use a good anti-perspirant deodorant under your arms. Remember also to clean your face daily to remove grime and dirt that builds up in your pores.

Don't neglect your teeth either! They are an important part of your health and need to be brushed and flossed daily to remove plaque and prevent bad breath.

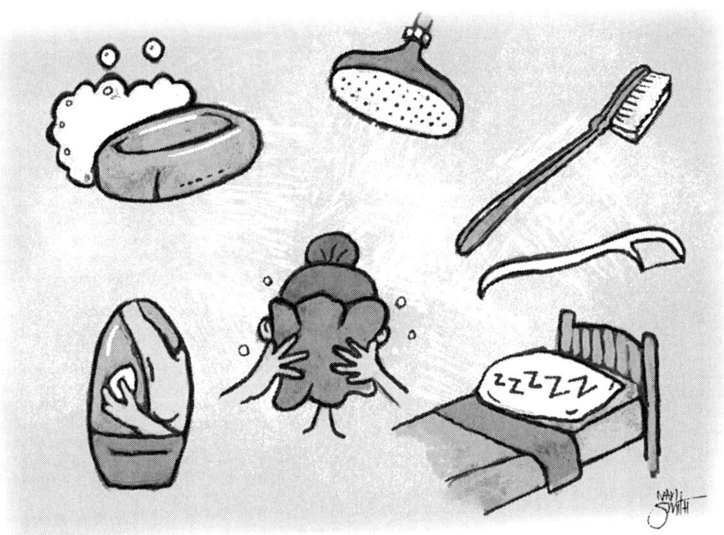

HEALTHY TOOLS

look after yourself

Imagine you have finally purchased your dream car. Shiny at first. A thing of beauty.

You drive it around with pride and visit all your friends. You cannot, however, be bothered washing it, so a mountain of dirt and grease builds up over the first year. You drive and drive the car, but you forget to check the oil and water, not to mention not filling the tank with petrol.

How far do you think you would get? I can tell you now that it would not be long before your prized car would stop. It cannot continue to run without constant attention and good fuel.

Our bodies are a bit like cars. They need constant **FUEL** and **CARE** in order to keep them running at their optimum. I read once how we should look after our bodies because they are the only houses we have. We only get one body, so we really need to take the time to care for it.

Diet

Be mindful of your **DIET**. In these days of high junk food and processed foods, make sure you try and get at least three serves of fruit and vegetables per day. Likewise, our bodies are made up of more than 50 per cent water. This means that we need to ensure we replace our fluids constantly. Two litres (eight glasses) of water per day is recommended.

Try filling a 1.5 litre plastic bottle with water at the beginning of the day. Carry this bottle around with you and drink from it wherever you go. If this sounds too much, fill a smaller bottle regularly throughout the day. If water is too boring for you, cut a small slice of lemon or lime and pop it in the bottle.

exercise

...away from the screen

Keep your body **HEALTHY** by making sure you exercise it regularly.

It's important to remember that exercise doesn't have to be a chore or something to dread. There are so many ways you can be physically active that can be enjoyable and even social. Joining a sports team, taking a dance class, going for a hike with friends, or even just taking a brisk walk around the neighbourhood can all be great options.

Remember that **CONSISTENCY** is key when it comes to exercise. Rather than trying to do an intense workout occasionally, aiming for regular, moderate exercise is more effective for overall health and well-being. So, whether it's 30 minutes of activity each day or a few longer workouts each week, finding a routine that works for you and sticking to it can have significant benefits for both physical and mental health.

Get active to keep the blood pumping around your body.

Some ideas:

- Walk the dog (or somebody else's)
- Take up a sport, e.g. netball, baseball, soccer
- Go for a run
- Go for a bushwalk with friends
- Take an aerobics class
- Join the local gym
- Rowing/canoeing
- Calisthenics
- Dancing
- Gymnastics
- Boxing
- Wrestling

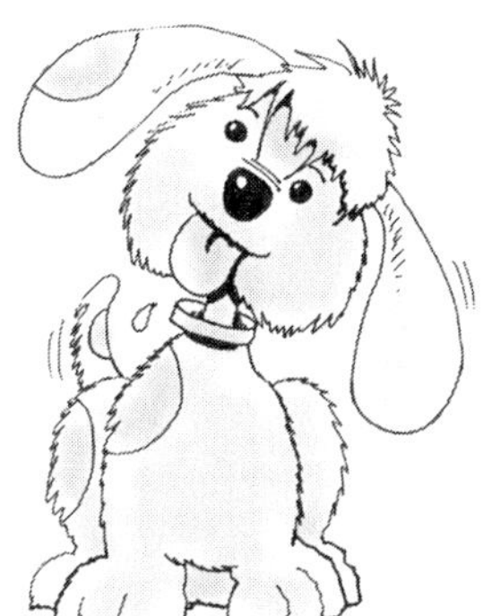

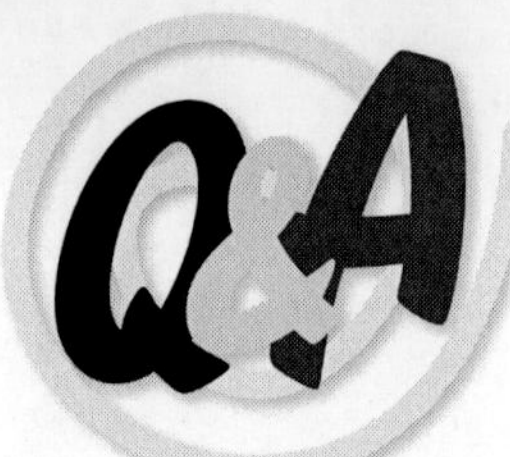

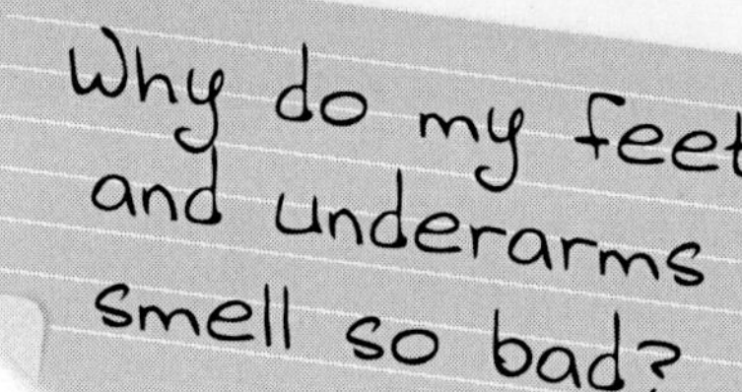

When we sweat,
our bodies are removing toxins from our bodies. That's why sweat doesn't particularly smell so good. Try and wear loose fitting cotton clothes, especially T-shirts that breath. This allows the sweat to move away from your body quickly.

How often should I shower?

Showering regularly is important as it gets rid of dead skin cells and the build-up of dirt and grease that comes from the air and the environment in which we are in each day. Showering daily is important — some girls even like to shower twice daily when they have their periods.

Skin condition?

Your skin is an important part of your body. When your skin is clear and healthy, you look great and in turn, feel better about yourself.

We often inherit our skin type fr parents. For example, if you hav olive (darker) complexion, usual one or both of your parents will have a similar skin type. Some girls have a paler skin type which is more prone to getting sunburnt. Whatever skin type you have, remember to take good care of it, just like you would any other part of your body.

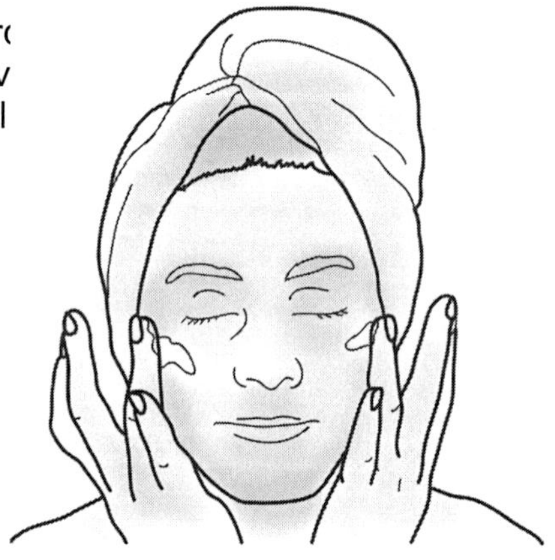

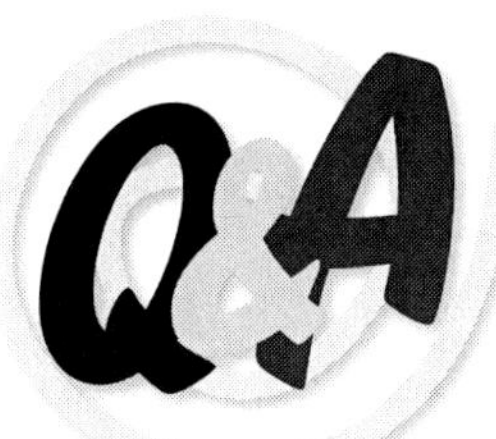

How do I get rid of the redness of my pimples?

There are many treatments that are available to help with pimples and acne. Talk to your pharmacy staff, who will be able to guide you towards the best form of action. Having pimples and severe acne can be one of the difficult stages of adolescence. Try and keep your skin as clean as possible. The good news is that it should get better as you get older.

Why do all the famous celebrities look like they all have fantastic skin? ... mine never looks that great!

The truth is, many don't! Many movie stars and models actually have poor skin, just like the rest of us. They may suffer from really oily or dry skin or have severe acne. In their case, however, they have access to professional photographers, and makeup artists who are paid to make sure that we can't notice these skin 'flaws'. If you think the celebrities have great skin, they have done their job well!

And with social media, and a vast range of filters available, most celebrities will not be posting natural images of themselves.

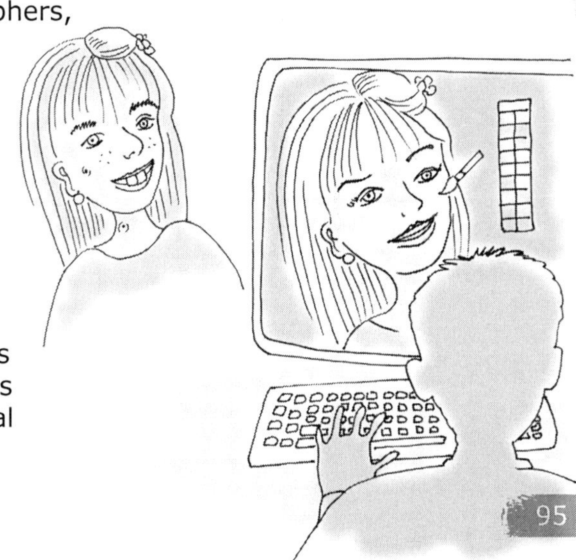

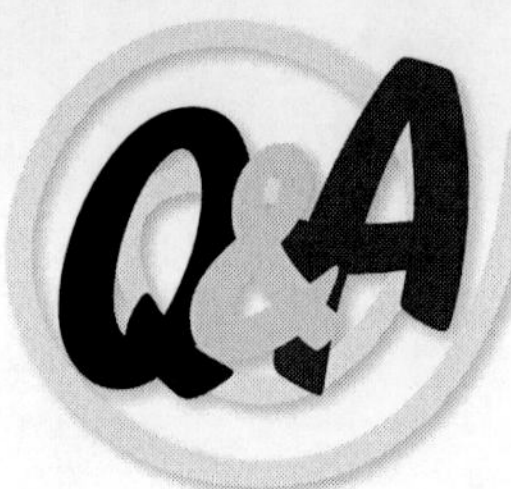

How can I prevent pimples?

Pimples are, unfortunately, quite often just a part of puberty. An increase in hormones running through the body can contribute to these nasty little critters, as well as our diet. Try using a good cleanser each evening — available from your local pharmacy — to clean your pores and get rid of any bacteria or dirt that can get stuck in them. You can also try washing your face in warm soapy water each evening, and avoid using too much makeup.

Is there anything wrong with me getting a fake tan?

Fake tans or skin lotions that turn our skin a shade of brown (or orange) seem to be quite okay medically, although I certainly wouldn't want to get in the habit of applying all that gunk to my skin unnecessarily all the time. Tanning lotion is a bit like cosmetic makeup: It can give you a bit of a pick-me-up if you are feeling a bit down, and can give your skin the appearance of a healthy glow. But treat all skin treatments like this in moderation. Don't become obsessed with it and forget who you really are!

sun care

When I was a teenager, I would cover my entire body in tanning oil and lie in the sun with my girlfriends on the beach while we baked ourselves silly. We would lay there for hours under the hot sun, then compare our tan marks until we got pretty burnt. I cringe now when I think of how stupid we were, but we know a lot more these days about the harmful affects of Ultra Violet rays and deliberately subjecting ourselves to the sun's harsh rays.

In our Western culture, skin cancer is very real and a silent and deadly killer. It is essential that you take skin care and prevention seriously. Do not assume that skin cancer affects only older people. Recently, a young girl of 25 was reported as having developed a skin melanoma. In her case, the cancer had reportedly spread throughout her body. Many young people die from skin-related cancer each year, so take it seriously.

Looking after your skin...

- *Drink lots of water.*
- *Eat lots of good foods, including fruits and vegetables.*
- *Participate in regular exercise.*
- *Make sure you get plenty of sleep.*
- *Always wear a SPF 35+ sunscreen when you are outside (you can get tinted moisturisers with a 35+ SPF protection).*
- *Wear a broad-brimmed type hat when you are under the sun to protect your ears and nose.*
- *Avoid wearing singlet tops under the sun to avoid burning your shoulders.*

Why do girls need to shave their legs and arm pits?

There is no set rule that says girls have to shave their legs and arm pits. In fact, in many cultures, girls do not shave at all and this is perfectly acceptable. In our Western society, it all comes down to your own personal choice: What works best for you! Many girls like to have clear, shaved skin on their legs and under their arms, but it is your choice: No one else's. Some girls prefer to keep the hair exactly as it grows and there is no medical reason why you should shave. Many girls feel more feminine when they shave, whereas guys like to be hairy because it is a sign of their manhood. For many, growing chest and underarm hair is a wonderfully obvious sign that they are becoming young men.

A word of caution here though: If you do decide to shave your legs or underarms, just remember that once you do begin this, the hair will generally grow back thicker and more quickly, so make sure you are certain of this choice. It's also a good idea to chat with a parent or adult first!

Why do some girls get their hair waxed?

Waxing is just another form of hair removal, although somewhat more painful and certainly not for the fainthearted. It hurts! This involves a warm wax being applied to the area of hair you want removed. Depending on the type of wax removal system, most commonly, a cloth is pressed down to join to the wax. Then, it is quickly ripped off, taking the wax and excess hair with it! ***OUCH!*** The benefits of waxing are that, generally speaking, the hair grows back at a slower pace because it is pulled out at the roots. ***(OUCH AGAIN!)***

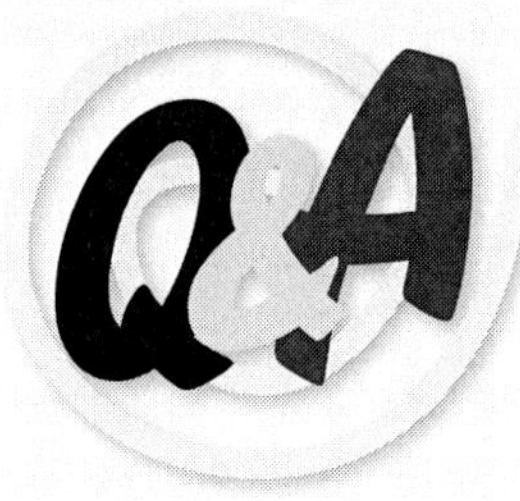

When should I start shaving my legs and underarms?

There is no set time – aside from obviously waiting until you well and truly have plenty of hair there to remove!

When I was about 14 years-old, one of my girlfriends came to stay for a weekend. We walked to the nearby supermarket, where she purchased some disposable razors to shave her legs. I had never done it before but I thought I would give it a go. The trouble is, once you start, you have to continue doing so, because the hair starts to grow back again.

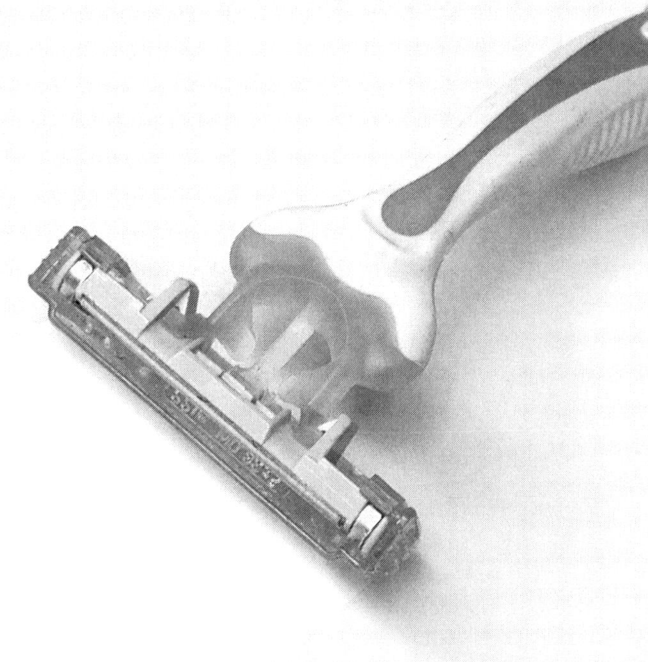

Sleep

Getting enough sleep is crucial in supporting your physical and mental health.

When I chat to young people about the topic of sleep, I find that generally, close to 80 per cent of them report that they have sleep issues – either trouble falling asleep or waking too early.

Remember, your body and brain are still developing, and quality sleep plays a significant role in this process. Sleep helps to repair and rejuvenate your body, boost your immune system, and promote healthy brain function, including memory, concentration, and mood regulation.

Not getting enough sleep can lead to a variety of negative consequences, including daytime sleepiness, irritability, difficulty focusing, and decreased academic performance. Additionally, sleep deprivation has been linked to an increased risk of mental health issues such as anxiety and depression. Therefore, it's important to prioritise getting the recommended amount of sleep each night to support your overall health and well-being.

You may find that you have trouble getting a good night's sleep. Between homework, extracurricular activities, and socialising with friends, it can be hard to find time to relax and wind down before bed. But one thing that may be keeping you up at night is your electronic devices.

Using electronic devices such as smartphones, tablets, and computers before bedtime can disrupt your sleep patterns and make it harder for you to fall asleep. Here are a few reasons why:

1. **Blue Light:**
   Electronic devices emit blue light, which can interfere with your body's production of melatonin, a hormone that regulates sleep. When you expose yourself to blue light before bedtime, your body thinks it's still daytime and may have trouble getting into sleep mode.

2. **Stimulating Content:**
   Using your devices before bed can also be mentally stimulating. Whether you're scrolling through social media or playing a video game, your brain may be too active to calm down and fall asleep.

3. **Interrupted Sleep:**
   If you keep your device close to you at night, you may be more likely to wake up if you receive a notification or message. This can interrupt your sleep and make it harder to get the rest you need.

A few tips to improve your sleep habits:

- Put your devices away at least an hour before bedtime. This will give your brain time to wind down and prepare for sleep.
- Use a traditional alarm clock instead of relying on your phone to wake you up in the morning. This will help you avoid the temptation to check your phone before bed or as soon as you wake up.
- Consider using the 'night mode' feature on your devices, which reduces the amount of blue light they emit. This can help reduce the impact on your sleep patterns.
- Charge your devices outside of your bedroom. This will help you avoid the temptation to check your phone or tablet when you should be sleeping.

By making these simple changes, you can improve your sleep habits and feel more rested and energised during the day. So, put down your devices before bedtime and give your brain the chance to relax and recharge.

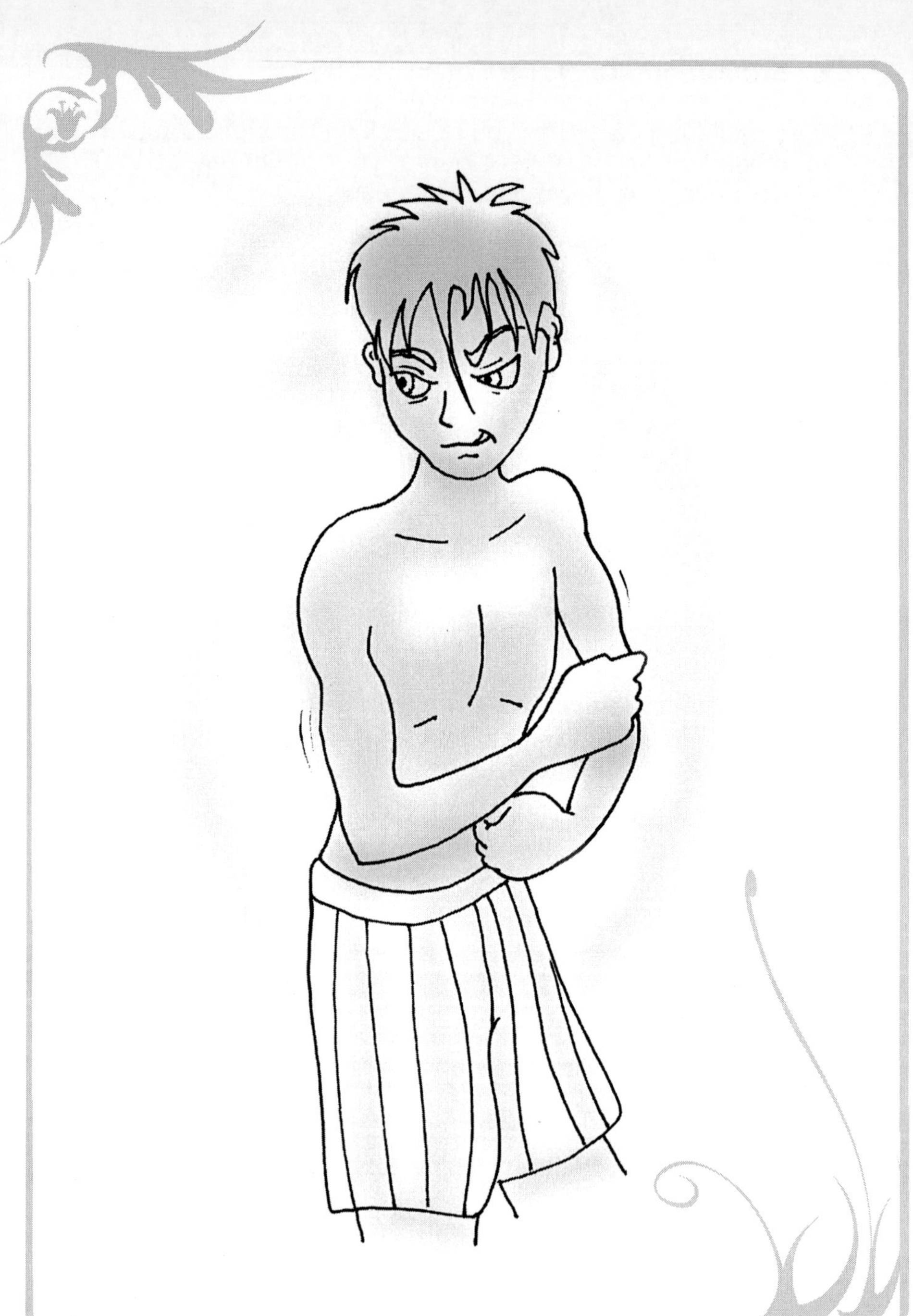

five//

secret boys' business

Parts of a boy's

Penis

One of the most important parts of the male reproductive system is the penis. The penis has three specific functions: Passing urine, passing semen (which contain the sperm; the cells that help to create a baby) and giving sexual pleasure. The long part of the penis is called the shaft, whilst the tip of the penis is called the glans, which is the most sensitive part.

The penis is made of spongy material and nerve endings. When a penis becomes erect, a surge of blood fills all the small chambers under the skin. This makes the penis hard and erect, which is needed if sexual intercourse is to take place between a man and a woman.

FACT: The penis cannot pass urine at the same time as semen. This is because during arousal, the urethra closes off so that urine cannot pass through at the same time as semen.

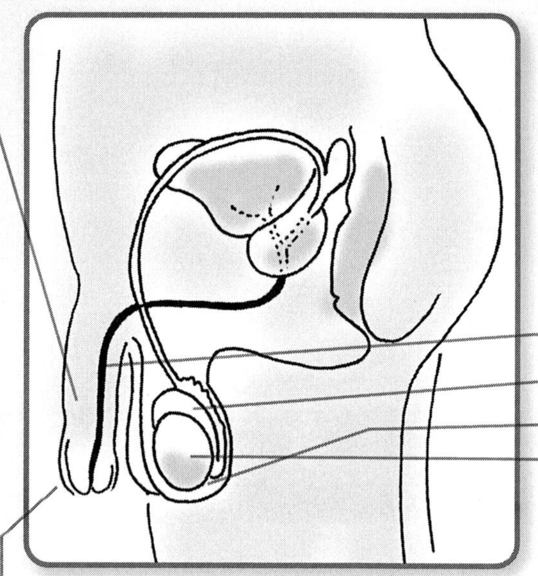

Foreskin

The foreskin is the skin right at the tip of the penis. The foreskin is only present in boys who have not been circumcised and covers the glans or tip of the penis. Some boys may have the tip of the foreskin removed at birth or soon after. This is called circumcision. It is not as common these days among many boys, however it still may be done for religious or cultural reasons. It is a reasonably small operation. Some parents have their boys circumcised because they feel that it is cleaner or the correct thing to do. In some instances, circumcisions may be performed in surgery out of medical necessity, such as when a boy gets an infection under the foreskin or does not practise good hygiene by cleaning himself properly.

Testicles (testes)

The main reproductive organs of the male body are the testicles, or testes, which produce sperm cells and also male hormones. The paired oval shaped testes (also known as gonads) are housed inside the scrotum. Quite often, the right teste can hang higher than the left one, so don't be too stressed if you notice this. Because sperm cells need just the right temperature to produce (about 3 degrees lower that your usual body temperature) the scrotum hangs outside the body.

Urethra

The Urethra is a thin tube found inside the penis, which passes urine from the bladder to the outside. This is also the same tube as semen travels through when you have an ejaculation, though it can never happen at the same time!

Epididymis

At the back of each testes is a cap formed by many, many long coils of tube called the epididymis. The function of the epididymis is to collect the immature sperm from the testes.

Scrotum

The scrotum is found under the penis and resembles a sack of skin that contains the testicles. The scrotum is an important part of sperm production because it controls the temperature of the testicles.

The testicles hang on the outside of the body so they can stay slightly cooler than the rest of the body. Sperm needs just the right conditions to be produced, and need to be produced in cooler conditions than the rest of the body.

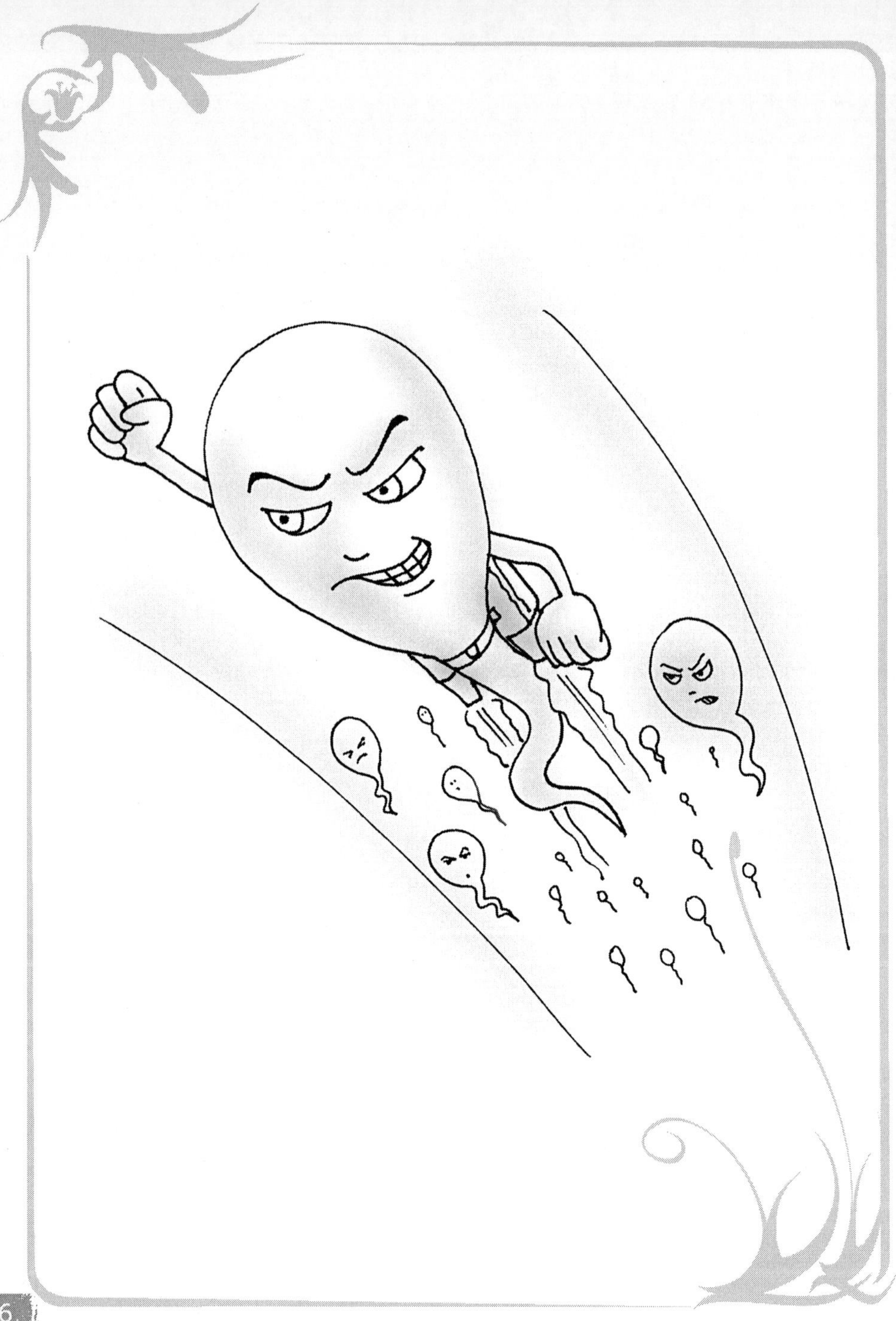

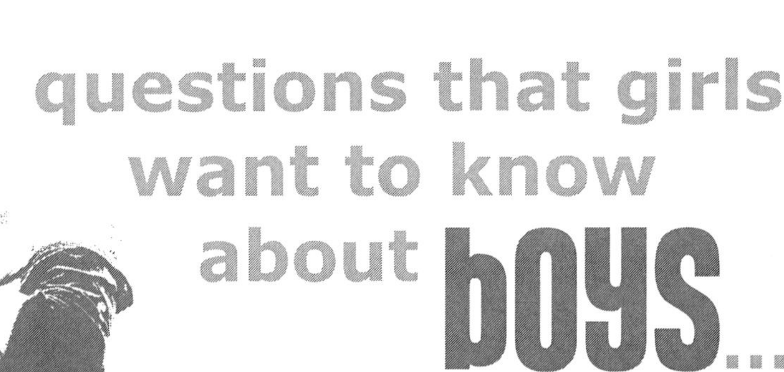

questions that girls want to know about boys...

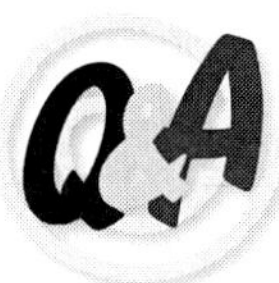

What is sperm?

Sperm are the male sex cells that contribute to a female's egg being fertilised to produce a baby.

Under a microscope, sperm look quite a lot like tadpoles. The sperm are produced inside the testicles of males, and mature in tubes called the **epididymis**. It's a bit like a mini factory that produces millions and millions of sperm every day once a boy begins puberty. Sperm move through a tube called the **vas** and mix with fluids that come from other glands.

Physical changes to boys during puberty...

- *Voice starts to change (squeaks and then deepens)*
- *Body starts to develop muscles, increase in weight*
- *Body shape begins to change*
- *Increase in height (growth spurt)*
- *Genitals increase in size*
- *Pubic hair begins to grow*
- *Sperm begins to develop*
- *Wet dreams may begin*

What is semen?

Semen is the fluid produced in males that contains sperm (the cells that are needed to fertilise an egg during intercourse). This fluid allows the sperm to easily travel out of the penis. The fluid contains proteins, enzymes and lubricants that provide nourishment for the sperm.

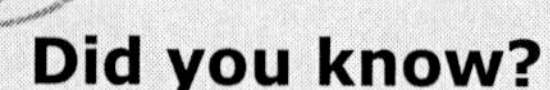

Did you know?

Sperm are cells and as such, are very prone to being damaged or killed! Sperm are sensitive to heat and extreme cold and can be damaged by extreme conditions. Poor sperm will never make the grade and will get left behind in the big race!

Why do boys get erections?

An **erection** is the term used when a boy's penis fills with blood through veins, allowing it to go stiff and erect. Because of this, erections are often referred to as 'stiffies' or 'boners'. A boy can get an erection for many different reasons; through stimulation or even from seeing or thinking about something that sexually excites him. The technical reason why a penis has been designed to go erect is so that it can enter a female's vagina during sexual intercourse.

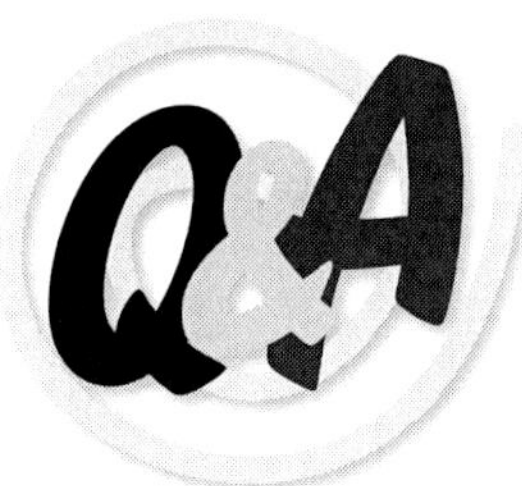

What is a 'wet dream'?

A **wet dream** is when semen comes out of the penis, usually when a boy is fast asleep. The term 'nocturnal emission' means occurring at night. This can be quite embarrassing for a guy when it happens, however it is nothing to worry about. It is all part of being a guy. If semen builds up in an adolescent boy's body, it sometimes needs to be released.

What is ejaculation?

Ejaculation is when semen exits the male's penis. This often occurs during intercourse, however, it can occur at other times, eg: during wet dreams.

Why do guys seem to only like skinny girls?

This is simply not true. Some girls actually believe that about many guys but the fact is, guys don't just like girls that are thin! In fact, guys are attracted to many other parts of a girl, not just her body size and shape. Your personality and character counts a lot for most guys so don't fool yourself into thinking you have to be any shape other than what you are!

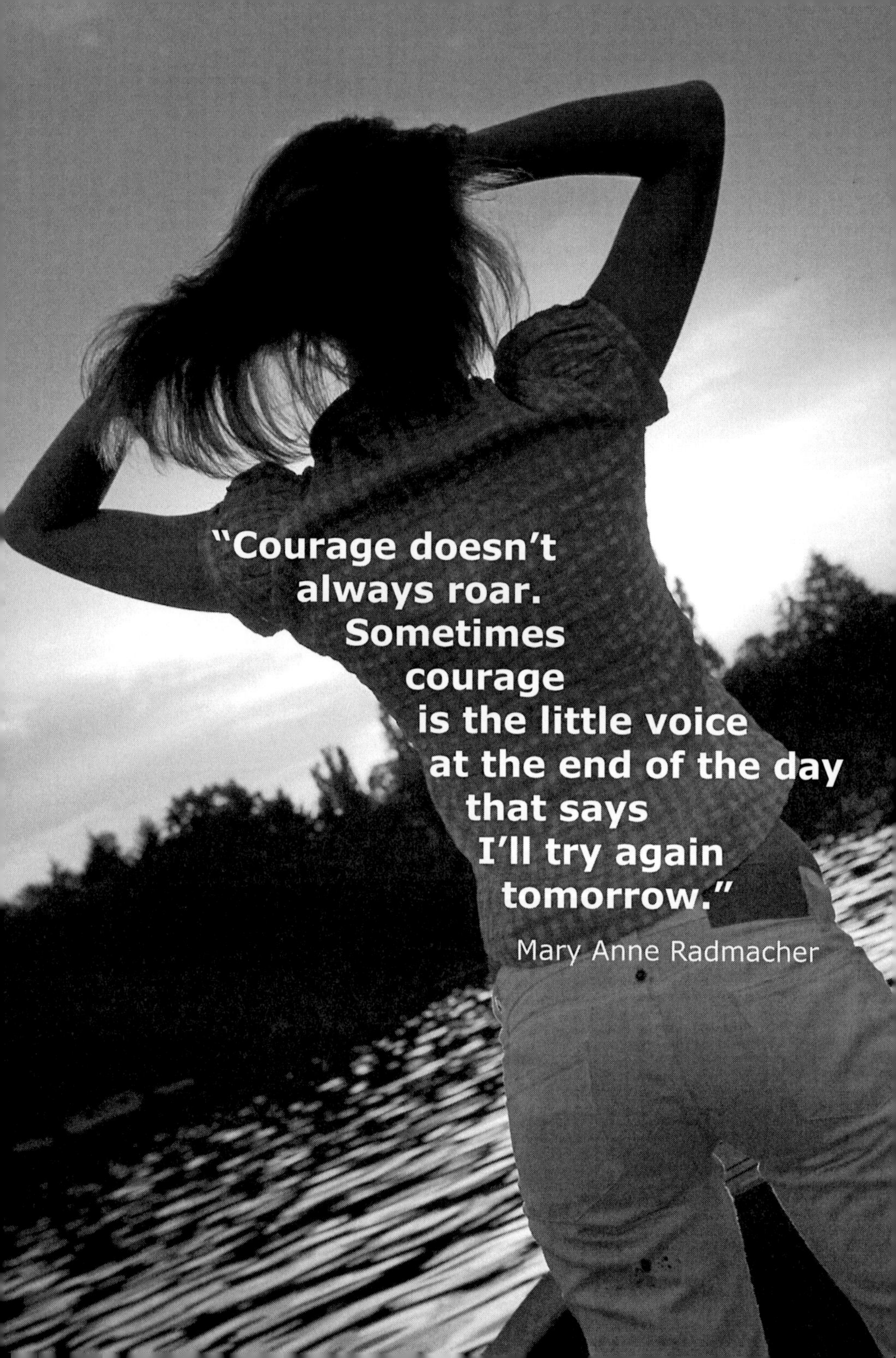
"Courage doesn't
always roar.
Sometimes
courage
is the little voice
at the end of the day
that says
I'll try again
tomorrow."
Mary Anne Radmacher

six//

the emotional roller coaster

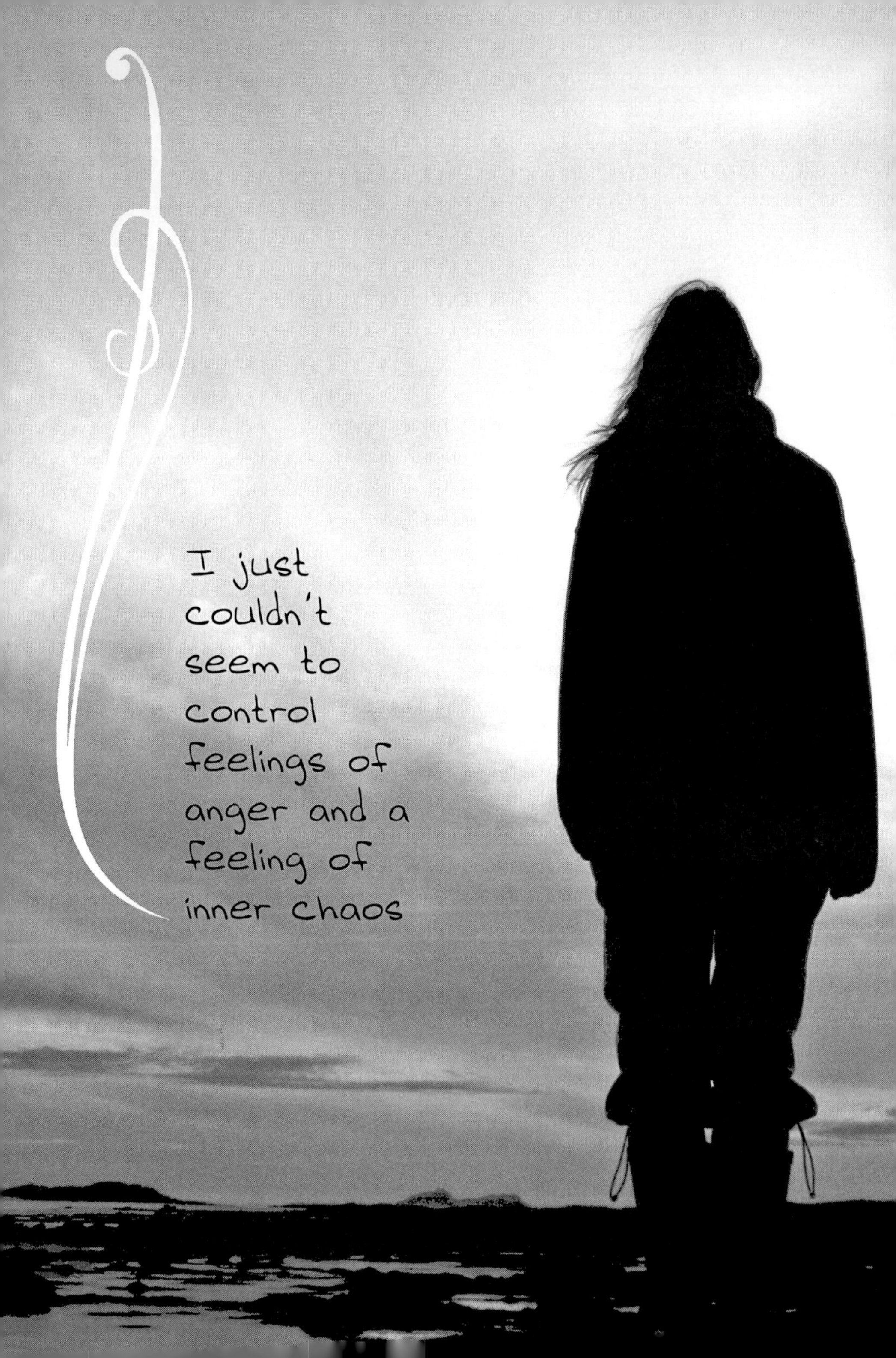
I just couldn't seem to control feelings of anger and a feeling of inner chaos

help me, I'm a wreck!

I hear you!

Of the thousands of teenage girls I have spoken with about being a teenager, this is by far the most common complaint. And no wonder! Our hormones (yes, there's that horrible word again) are totally running rampant in our bodies. It is during these delightful teenage years that we will find ourselves flying off the handle at everyone around us for no apparent reason. Whereas you used to love hanging out with your younger sister or brother, you now find yourself turning feral as soon as they dare to enter your bedroom! And your parents are by no means safe from these tirades. They may get yelled and screamed at just for asking how school was today, when not so long ago this perfectly normal type of question was acceptable and did not usually incur aggressive responses!

I recall when I was in secondary school, trying desperately to wade through my awful Maths homework. Mum would simply slide open my bedroom door and I would hurl a tirade of abuse about the horrors of school, life, Maths, my brother, teachers, etc! Usually, this was capped off by a flying Maths book aimed directly at the door! I often had mum in tears over my unnecessary outbursts of anger. I'd feel pretty awful afterwards but I just couldn't seem to control feelings of anger and a feeling of inner chaos.

It is during these delightful teenage years that we will find ourselves flying off the handle at everyone around us for no apparent reason.

my hormones are OUT OF CONTROL

☹ *I feel angry or frustrated for no real reason.*
☹ *I look ugly, feel ugly.*
☹ *I think I'm fat.*
☹ *I have no friends. No one really likes me.*
☹ *What's my purpose in life? Do I really matter?*
☹ *I don't feel like hanging out with anyone.*
☹ *I have no energy. I can't be bothered.*
☹ *I'm really, really tired!*
☹ *Don't anyone dare talk to me!*
☹ *I cannot concentrate!*
☹ *I'm exhausted!*
☹ *I have absolutely NO motivation!*
☹ *I feel like punching someone for no real reason.*

Do any of these feelings sound familiar to you?

Some people will rarely experience these 'out-of-control' feelings. Others will constantly feel like they are on a rollercoaster of emotions.

Do you ever have a day, or a series of days, when many of these thoughts are running through your head?

Well I can say that I have felt like that all in the same day, and it can often feel a bit like you're losing your mind. It really can! You can feel totally out of control and have no idea why. It can actually be quite scary as you lose all motivation and feel like life is just way too difficult.

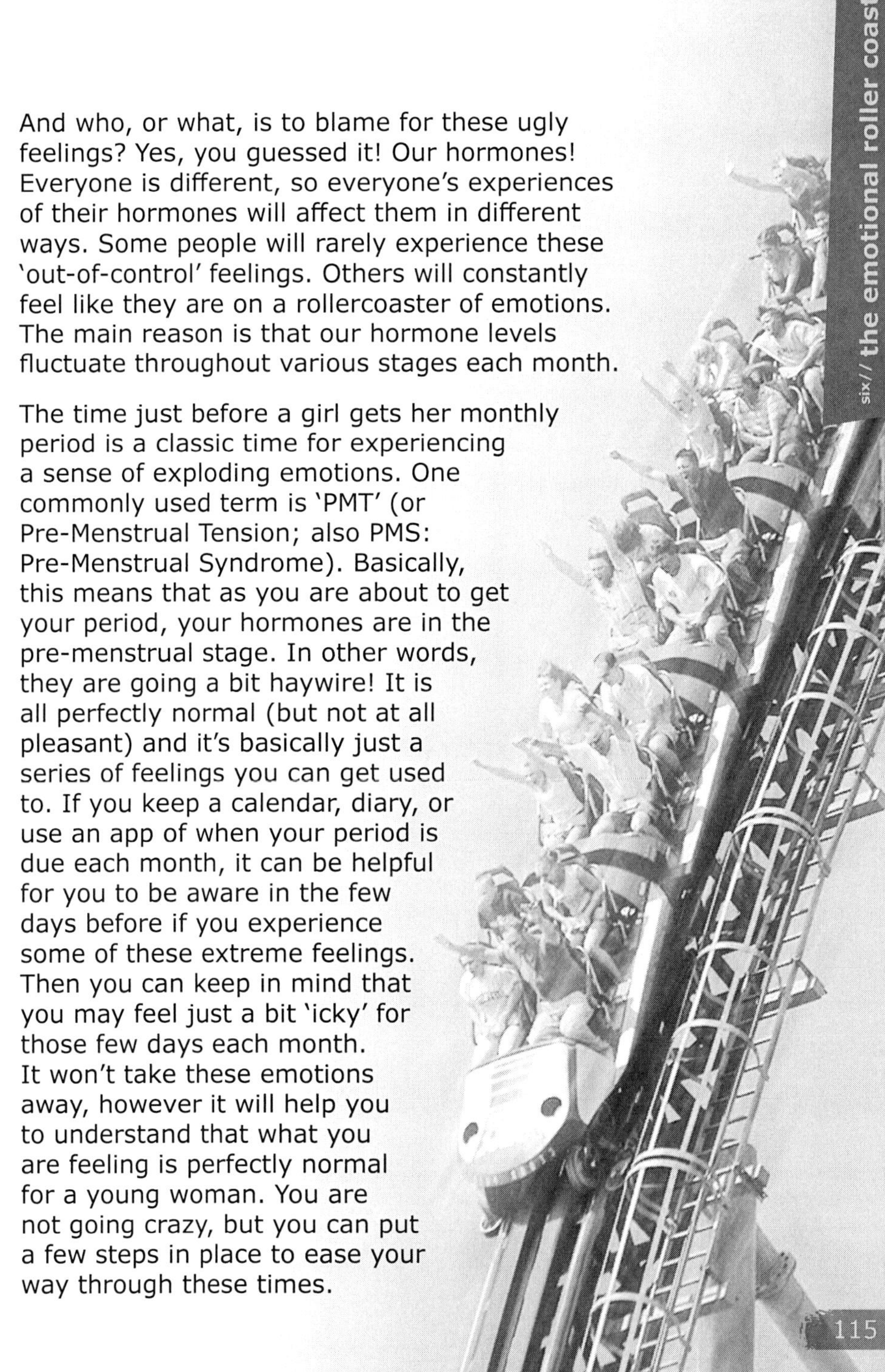

And who, or what, is to blame for these ugly feelings? Yes, you guessed it! Our hormones! Everyone is different, so everyone's experiences of their hormones will affect them in different ways. Some people will rarely experience these 'out-of-control' feelings. Others will constantly feel like they are on a rollercoaster of emotions. The main reason is that our hormone levels fluctuate throughout various stages each month.

The time just before a girl gets her monthly period is a classic time for experiencing a sense of exploding emotions. One commonly used term is 'PMT' (or Pre-Menstrual Tension; also PMS: Pre-Menstrual Syndrome). Basically, this means that as you are about to get your period, your hormones are in the pre-menstrual stage. In other words, they are going a bit haywire! It is all perfectly normal (but not at all pleasant) and it's basically just a series of feelings you can get used to. If you keep a calendar, diary, or use an app of when your period is due each month, it can be helpful for you to be aware in the few days before if you experience some of these extreme feelings. Then you can keep in mind that you may feel just a bit 'icky' for those few days each month. It won't take these emotions away, however it will help you to understand that what you are feeling is perfectly normal for a young woman. You are not going crazy, but you can put a few steps in place to ease your way through these times.

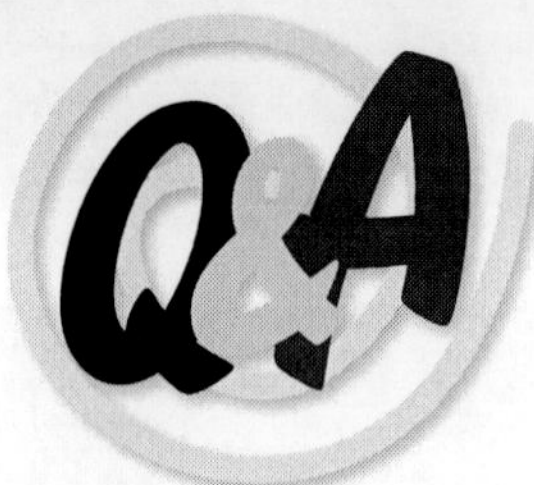

Why do I get grumpy sometimes, even when I haven't got my period?

Changes in your hormone levels, which can cause mood changes or grumpiness, often occurs during different stages of our monthly menstruation cycle. During different times each month, hormone levels in our body rise and fall, affecting our moods. Often, our diet can also affect our moods, so make sure you get plenty of vitamins and minerals in your system by eating plenty of fruits and vegetables.

Why do girls experience mood swings?

Mood swings occur for many reasons and often well before puberty even hits. Your hormones are most likely to blame, however family changes, pressures at school or lack of sleep can also affect your moods too. You can try recording on a calendar, or in your diary, the days when you feel especially moody or 'out of sorts'. If you can see a pattern developing after a few months, you could assume that, most likely, it will be the hormonal changes at work in your body. Having a chat with a trusted adult or your family doctor about this could also be helpful.

PMT experiences...

A collection of memories and anecdotes from girls and women who've survived their PMT experiences...

'About 2 to 3 days before I get my period, I can feel just awful. I feel totally unmotivated and a bit, well, just unhappy. I can't be bothered doing anything and my family just annoys me for no apparent reason. They can't say anything right and I find myself snapping at them easily. Then I feel bad later. The worst thing is that I often have no idea why I am feeling that way. Then, I get my period and it all makes sense!'

'When I'm experiencing the symptoms of PMT, I get lower back pain. I also cry at the smallest and most trivial things, but at the same time those emotions seem so real and significant to me. And anyone who brushes me off as "Pre Menstrual" in those crucial moments is not a popular person that day! I also get really sore boobs! Running and tight, squeezy hugs are not a happening thing for a good few days!'

'It's amazing how many girls feel better if they exercise when they are experiencing the symptoms of PMT. It doesn't have to be overly strenuous but I'm pretty sure there's a scientific reason for us feeling better after exercise. I know that it personally worked for me. I didn't feel like doing anything, but once I began exercising, I felt it made a huge difference.'

'When you've got PMT, crying really does help! It's biologically good for you! So go get a movie that gives you a good reason to have a really good sook. It's an effective way to release all that inner frustration and emotion without hurting the people around you!'

beating the pmt blues...

- *Spend some quality time by yourself. Watch your favourite movie.*
- *Run a beautiful hot bubble bath for yourself, light some scented candles and take a good book or magazine with you!*
- *Sleep in!*
- *Pick flowers.*
- *Laugh out loud.*
- *Have a really good cry (watch a real soppy movie and let it all out with a big box of Kleenex!).*
- *Ask for cuddles.*
- *Write in your diary (if you keep one) about how you are feeling. (Verbalising it or actually writing it down can really help!)*
- *Try cardmaking or something else creative that you enjoy.*
- *Call a girlfriend who you haven't spoken to in ages.*
- *Go to the supermarket and buy your favourite junk food — chocolate, chips, anything you feel like, as long as it's comfort food. Don't worry about the fat content today. Just go home and enjoy it with a good movie!*
- *Spend the day at the shops. Window shopping can be a great time-waster and can just make you feel better.*
- *Go for a really long walk and just clear your head and thoughts. You'll feel heaps better.*
- *Sleep!*
- *Paint your fingernails & toenails.*

A word of caution... don't make any major decisions, such as completely changing your hair style, or leaving home, when you are experiencing pre-menstrual hormones! Things often seem a lot worse when your hormones are going crazy!

seven//

Focus on friends

FRIENDSHIPS

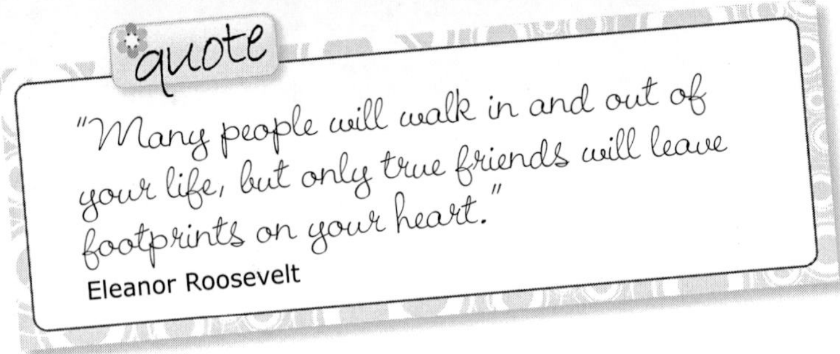

Where would we be without **FRIENDS**? Our relationships with friends and mates can be some of the most special, unique, and influential aspects of our lives. Many young people agree that their friendships are a very important part of their lives. They just wouldn't cope as well through all the changes and hassles of adolescence without such support.

Have you ever noticed that people who are constantly surrounded by friends are the friendliest towards others?

As I write this chapter, one of my dear friends has just left after having lunch at my place. We have been friends for many years now, which is amazing, since we became friends when we were teaching at the same school. The thing I appreciate about her is that she has always been my friend and accepted me for all that I am. If we don't speak to each other for a while because of the busyness of our lives, it's okay. We know that our friendship is lifelong.

Throughout your teen years, your friendships will most likely alternate and change. Some friendships may remain for life; however, some won't. And that's okay.

Friendships can also be seasonal. In primary school, for example, we may have a couple of important friends whom we think will be our very best friends forever. Then we may move on and go to separate high schools and lose touch with these friends. We may then make new friends in high school, then university or work, and so on.

Friendships are absolute gifts. They can be unique and special and certainly help us get through the happy and difficult seasons of our lives. Real friends are different from the variety of people you will meet throughout your life and be friendly with (acquaintances). Real friendships are built on honesty and a solid relationship of trust. They stand the test of time.

You may only have a small handful of truly good friends throughout your life. Two of my dearest friends are from my latter high school years (now 37-year friendships), whilst most recent friendships have developed in my working life and through relationships I have developed with other mums. Another important friendship is from my teen years. That relationship has stood the test of time as we have experienced joys and tragedies together.

If you want great friendships, you must first be a good friend. And if you want more friends, be one to others.

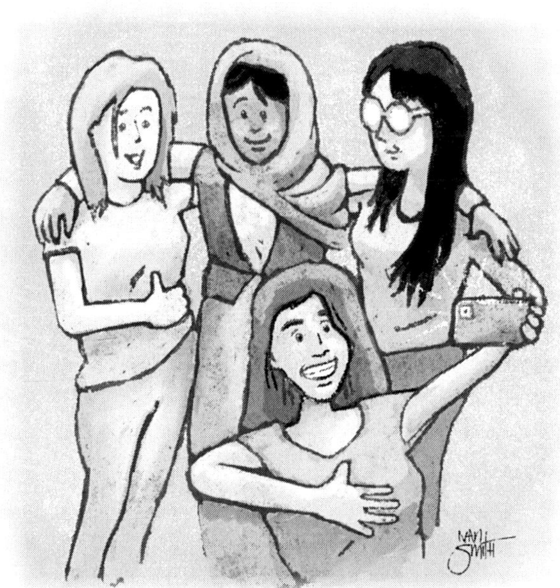

finding calm in conflict

Conflicts are a normal part of being in a community, but they can be tricky to handle. Dealing with conflict in a healthy way takes practice.

Remember, your teen brain is still under construction and your emotional intelligence and communication skills are still developing.

When dealing with conflict:

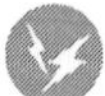

Identify the Problem

The first step in resolving any conflict is to try to identify the underlying issue. This may involve acknowledging your own feelings and perspective, as well as those of the other person.

As yourself questions like:

"What am I feeling?"

"What does the other person seem to be feeling?"

"What might be going on for them?"

Active Listening

This means paying close attention to what the other person is saying. This can be tricky when we are right in the thick of a conversation as our mind can be busy thinking how we want to respond.

Listen without interrupting (you'll get the chance to have your say).

Show empathy and understanding by repeating back what you've heard the other person say and ask clarifying questions to ensure you understand their perspective.

Express your feelings

Once you've taken the time to listen to the other person, it's important to take the time to express your own feelings and perspective about the issue.

Use 'I' statements to communicate your point of view, rather than placing blame on the other person. For example, instead of saying "You're wrong!" try saying:

"I feel upset when this happens" or
"This is not how I understand the situation."

Better together

Try and work together to find a solution. When both parties have had the opportunity to express their feelings and experience, it is time to work together to find a solution. It may involve compromise, and negotiation until you both find a solution that feels comfortable and peaceful for both of you. You may find that you have differing opinions on a particular issue, and that may mean that you find a respectful boundary. Perhaps you will not agree but learn to understand and value each other's ideas and opinions.

Sometimes, you may need to create some space between you – for a time. This can give both of you some valuable time to retreat, reflect and find calm during conflict.

Talk to a helpful adult

Dealing with conflict and hurt feelings can be a tricky business when you are a teenager. However, this is a life skill that you will practice time and time again in your adolescent years, as you move into adulthood.

There may be times when you need extra assistance to navigate a difficult situation. This is where a helpful adult can provide extra support and guidance. Reach out to a parent, carer, teacher, or other adult you trust.

By listening, expressing your feelings, communicating effectively, and working together to find a solution, you can improve your relationships and build positive connections with others.

What to do if...

quote

"A true friend should never pressure you into doing something that makes you feel uncomfortable." Unknown

During my late teens, one of my best friends was having a group of friends over one night. He attended a different school to me; however, we had forged a friendship through living close to each other. His friends also attended a high-profile private school.

That evening, the group lit up a bong with marijuana. It was my first sight of drug use. I admit I had sometimes smoked cigarettes on a social basis but had made the choice long before then that I would not take drugs.

That night, I was offered a smoke of dope by my best friend, but politely declined.

"I'm just happy to smoke one of my cigarettes," I replied. "Are you sure?" he responded. "Yep, absolutely."

That was that! No pressure, no snide remarks about being a 'wuss' or 'lame.' I felt completely at ease. He was a true friend who just loved me for me and valued our friendship beyond anything, including drugs.

There are going to be many instances over your teen years, and beyond, where you are going to be faced with pressures to do things that are not in your best interest. This is often referred to as 'peer pressure.' When you are surrounded by peers who engage in certain behaviours, hold certain beliefs, or are engaging in risk-taking behaviour, you will have to decide what you are going to do. You will be faced with a myriad of decisions over your life. Some of your choices will come down to the values you hold, and the personal choices you want to make for your mind and body.

personal POLiCY

In the above example, I had already decided that my personal policy was I would never partake in illicit drugs. I had already made that decision for myself. So, when I was in the position of being offered a drug, I could very clearly say "no thanks."

There will be many decisions you will have to make in your teen, and future years; it is helpful to think about your standpoint on a range of issues you may face relating to drugs, alcohol, engaging in sexual conduct, relationships and dating, online behaviour, and more.

If you take the time now to think about your viewpoint on these areas, it will help you when faced with those important decisions.

I encourage you to take some time and write down your person policies in the space provided on the following page. You don't have to write them all now. Come back to this page when you again when you are faced with a situation or decision.

THOUGHTS ON... GOSSIP

"Don't waste your time with explanations: people only hear what they want to hear."
Paulo Coelho

"Watch the way you talk. Let nothing foul or dirty come out of your mouth. Say only what helps, each word a gift."
Ephesians 4:29 (The Message)

"The only time people dislike gossip is when you gossip about them."
Will Rogers

"Don't be bluffed into silence by the threats of bullies. There's nothing they can do to your soul, your core being."
Matthew 10:28a (The Message)

"Words kill, words give life; they're either poison or fruit – you choose."
Proverbs 18:21 (The Message)

"Strong minds discuss ideas, average minds discuss events, weak minds discuss people."
Socrates

"Isn't it kind of silly to think that tearing someone else down builds you up?"
Sean Covey

when a friendship is UNHEALTHY

Unhealthy friendships can feel a bit like a vacuum cleaner sucking all the energy out of you. It's all heading one way!

In other words, unhealthy friendships are one sided — that is, one person is always doing the work and having to help the other one. Whilst it is true that all friendships will be tested at times, and may go through difficulties at certain points in your lives, it is important to remember that it is just like a partnership. It needs to work for both of you.

Needy friends can be quite difficult – the friend who has a low self-image and is always complaining about being 'too fat' or 'too ugly'... There is only a certain amount of this that people can take. My advice here is simple... be a good friend yourself. Affirm your friends, reminding them that they are important and worthwhile people.

On the issue of body shape and size, it's a good idea to not get caught in that battle. Of course, if you are worried about a friend's health, make sure you tell an adult. Otherwise, try to ignore negative behaviour as it will only seek to bring ***you*** down, and ***you*** don't need that.

If you have a friend or peer who is into things that you know are just wrong and not okay... **RUN A MILE!!!** If such a person is a close friend, of course this can be difficult, because you don't want to abandon a person making unhealthy choices. But don't nurture a friendship with someone who is making a deliberate choice to do dangerous or unhealthy things.

I have been fortunate in my life that I have always been drawn to positive and encouraging people as friends. I have nurtured friendships with those people who have similar qualities and attitudes to me. You will find that most people you develop friendships with happen because you share similar beliefs or interests.

dealing with BULLYING

Bullying is a serious issue that affects many teenagers. It can take many different forms, such as physical, verbal, or online harassment. Bullying can cause emotional distress and have long-term effects on the victim's mental health, including anxiety and depression.

The main characteristic of bullying is the power imbalance between the bully and the victim. The bully uses their power to control and intimidate the victim, often with the intention of causing harm. Bullies may also be motivated by a desire to fit in with their peers or gain social status.

It's important to understand that bullying is not the victim's fault. No one deserves to be bullied, and it's never okay to blame the victim for what is happening to them. If you or someone you know is being bullied, it's essential to seek help and support from a trusted adult, such as a teacher, parent, or counsellor.

A few years ago, I saw a woman on an American talk show complaining how she could not move forward in her life. She explained how she had suffered immense emotional and verbal bullying 20 years prior. The culprit had been a fellow female student at her high school. The victim had become pregnant as a teenager and copped a great deal of verbal abuse especially by one 'popular and attractive' girl. Both women were re-united on the show in front of a studio audience.

The victim, to that day, was devastated by the childhood bullying.

She had carried around a burden of rejection and hurt for two decades.

The most frightening thing was the reaction of the alleged bully. She claimed she had no recollection of the girl on stage or of the verbal attacks she had made.

She apologised but remained incredulous at the degree of hurt.

Signs of Bullying

Bullying can be difficult to identify, especially if it's happening online or behind closed doors. However, there are some common signs that may indicate that someone is being bullied:

- Physical injuries, such as bruises, cuts, or scratches
- Changes in behaviour, such as becoming withdrawn or anxious
- Loss of interest in activities they used to enjoy
- Difficulty sleeping or nightmares
- Declining grades or academic performance
- Avoidance of school or social situations
- Unexplained absences from school or activities

If you notice any of these signs in yourself or someone you know, it's important to act and seek help.

Dealing with Bullying

If you are being bullied, it's important to remember that you are not alone. There are people who can help you, and there are steps you can take to protect yourself:

Speak up
It can be challenging to speak up about bullying, but it's essential to tell someone you trust. This could be a teacher, counsellor, parent, or friend.

Stay calm
Bullies often try to get a reaction out of their victims, so it's essential to stay calm and avoid reacting emotionally. Try to remain composed and respond in a non-confrontational way.

Document the bullying
Keep a record of any incidents of bullying, including the date, time, and what happened. This can be useful if you need to report the bullying to someone in authority.

Avoid retaliation
It may be tempting to retaliate against a bully, but this can escalate the situation and make things worse. Instead, focus on staying safe and seeking help.

Take care of yourself
Bullying can take a toll on your mental health, so it's important to take care of yourself. Make sure to eat healthily, exercise, and engage in activities you enjoy.

Preventing Bullying

Preventing bullying is everyone's responsibility.
Here are some things you can do to help **PREVENT** bullying:

Speak out against bullying
If you witness bullying, speak out against it. Let the bully know that their behaviour is not acceptable.

Be kind
Small acts of kindness can go a long way in preventing bullying. Make an effort to be friendly and inclusive to others.

Stand up for others
If you see someone being bullied, stand up for them. Let them know that they are not alone.

Get involved
Join a club or organisation that focuses on preventing bullying, such as a peer counselling group or anti-bullying club.

Educate yourself
Learn more about bullying and its effects. The more you know, the better equipped you'll be to prevent it.

your tongue, a sword?

quote

"Watch the way you talk. Let nothing foul or dirty come out of your mouth. Say only what helps, each word a gift."
Ephesians 4:29 (The Message)

Name-calling is bullying. You know the expression, "Sticks and stones may break my bones, but words will never harm me"? What a load of garbage!

I can vividly recall verbal bullying, way back as a 12-year-old, in Year 7. I have always been someone of small stature and was easily the smallest in my class back then. One fellow student came up with the nickname 'weasel' for me. I absolutely hated that. It made me feel like some awful little animal. Why couldn't they think up a title like 'little cutie' or something like that? Well, I coped reasonably well, until the last day of the school year when our class teacher was giving out Christmas cards. They were lovely hand-made cards with a caricature of ourselves on the front. As mine came around, I couldn't believe my eyes; right there above my very cute portrait was the word 'weasel'! I couldn't believe that even my teacher had picked up on that name!

Well, I am still small in stature, but I don't let it bother me.

I tell this story to illustrate, though, that names 'stick'! Some 30 years later, I can still recall that experience as though it was yesterday.

>>>

You may be a person who occasionally calls people names, for whatever reason. You need to understand that the words that come out of your mouth can have a lasting effect on someone, though you may not think so at the time. You may say, "Oh, but they know that I am only joking." Well, they may say that, but words have a way of sticking in our minds if they are offensive or hurtful. And they can replay themselves repeatedly like a recording in our minds for as long as we allow them to. So please, remember that your tongue is a very powerful weapon, even though you may not physically hurt someone… you may cause even greater emotional damage.

You need to make sure that the words that come out of your mouth will not cause someone else to feel bad. Use your words to build others up, not destroy their self-image.

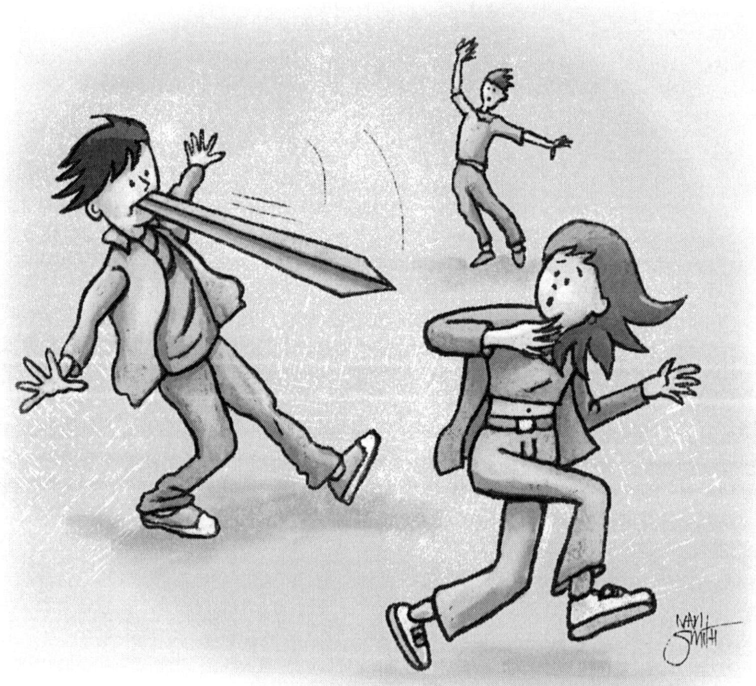

dealing with MUD SLINGERS

Don't allow those hurtful words to stick!

Throughout your teen years and beyond, you will most likely encounter negative or nasty comments directed at you or around you. Why? Because you are dealing with humans and let's face it – all of us can be guilty of having a negative attitude at times, and likewise, can say negative or hurtful things to others in the heat of the moment.

I recall one day when I was a teenager, having a conversation with an acquaintance – let's just say that we had a difference of opinion at the time. It wasn't going in a particularly positive direction, when completely out of the blue, this person said something incredible hurtful and potentially destructive to me. So much so that in the moment I felt like I'd been literally punched in the guts – it momentarily took my breath away.

Now, in my **HEART**, I knew without doubt that what this person said was completely false – however, my mind and body recoiled in shock.

So, what did I do next?

1. **SUIT UP**
   I want you to imagine that you are wearing a suit that is made from Teflon fabric (Teflon is that non-stick surface they coat fry pans with). You can make your suit any colour you wish, the point is – **NOTHING** sticks to your Teflon Suit.

2. **LET THE MUD SLIDE OFF**
   When I had that nasty comment flung at me like a giant pile of wet, sticky mud – I imagined that it hit my bright suit and then just oozed all the way to the ground, and then I stepped away from it. I did not let it stick. >>>

Negative and hurtful comments can only have power if we allow them to stick to us. They are only words – and words have no power if reject them.

WE get to decide if we want to take a nasty comment on board and let it affect us.

WE get to choose our response.

That is a powerful thing.

3. **DON'T BE A MUD SLINGER**
   When we are the recipient of nasty words or comments, it is easy for us to go straight into defence mode. We've just been hit! (metaphorically) and our immediate reaction can be to retaliate.

   It's important to remember that hurtful comments or actions from others are most often a reflection of their own internal struggles, rather than a true reflection of who we are as individuals. It can be tempting to respond defensively, however, by taking a step back and recognising that the person is likely hurting, can help us respond with empathy. It doesn't excuse their behaviour – they will have to own that for themselves, but it does help us flick the mud to the ground.

4. **SPEAK UP WHEN YOU SEE MUD BEING SLUNG**
   It takes courage to speak up when you see mud being slung at another person. Others, in that situation, would appreciate some help. I'm quite certain that they'd hope a friend or bystander would speak out on their behalf and let the mudslinger know that it is not okay to be unkind or hurtful.

   You may check in with the person affected and let them know that you see what happened and you are there for them.

   If it is bullying situation, and it's a repeated action, consider offering to accompany them to the school counsellor or welfare support person.

   By remembering that hurt people, hurt people, we can begin to break the cycle of negativity and work towards building more compassionate and supportive relationships with those around us.

thoughts on friends

'Friendship consists in forgetting what one gives, and remembering what one receives.'
Alexandre Dumas (1803-1870, French novelist)

'You can always tell a real friend. When you've made a fool of yourself, he doesn't feel you've done a permanent job.'
Laurence J Peter, Canadian writer

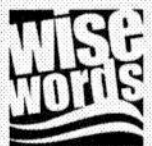

'A friend is always loyal.'

Proverbs 17:17a NLT

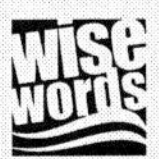

'Friends come and friends go, but a true friend sticks by you like family.'

Proverbs 18:24 The Message

'True happiness consists not in the multitude of friends but in the worth and choice.'
Ben Jonson (1573-1637), English dramatist and poet

'Never refuse any advance of friendship, for if nine out of ten bring you nothing, one alone may repay you.'
Madame de Tencin

'I have learned that to have a good friend is the purest of all God's gifts for it is a love that has no exchange or payment.'
Frances Farmer (1910-1970), American actress & writer

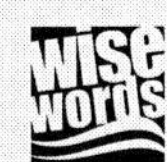

'There is no greater love than to lay down one's life for one's friends.'

John 15:13 NLT

'The antidote for 50 enemies is one friend.'
Aristotle (384-322 BC), Greek philosopher

'It is one of the blessings of friends that you can afford to be stupid with them.'
Ralph Waldo Emerson (1803-1882), American essayist & philosopher

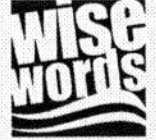

'Do a favour and win a friend forever; nothing can untie that bond.'

Proverbs 18:19 The Message

'The only way to have a friend is to be one.'
Ralph Waldo Emerson (1803-1882), American essayist & philosopher

'The proper office of a friend is to side with you when you are wrong. Nearly anybody will side with you when you are in the right.'
Mark Twain (1835-1910), American writer

'Friendship with oneself is all important because without it, one cannot be friends with anyone else in the world.'
Eleanor Roosevelt (1884-1962), First Lady of the USA

Gossiping is something wrong, something bad.
If you spread secrets, the person who it's about
Will have a permanent scar
They will never be able to totally forget about it.
This person can't talk to her friends any more
Because they have hurt her too many times.

Are you one of the friends?
Do you treat your friends this way?
Well if you are, you need to know,
It's not the right way to treat your friends.
Soon it won't be a problem though,
Because you won't have any friends left.

By Taylor Dykstra

eight//

taming the gossip dragon

gossip

sticks and stones ... really *do* hurt as much as words

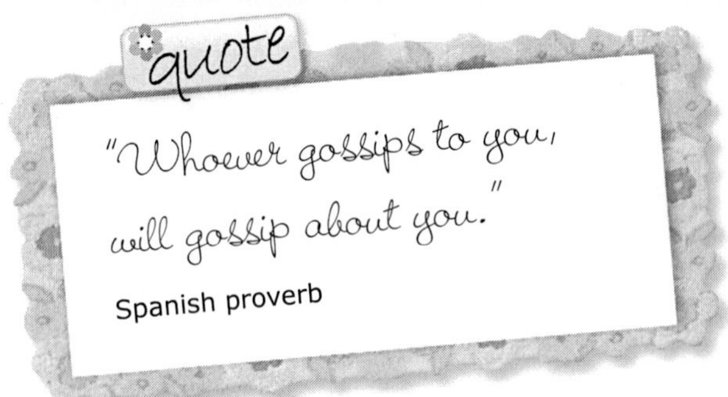

GOSSIPING and **NASTINESS** can be one of the most difficult parts of being a young person.

A definition I use for 'gossip' is anything said that you wouldn't be perfectly happy to say in front of the person involved.

But, more importantly, the effect is longer-lasting than the time it takes for the comment to be made.

Gossiping can be one of the most soul-destroying things a person can experience. Lighting a match in the middle of a forest. At first, only a few small twigs are lit, and a small flame grows, then that flame catches onto another branch and before you know it, the whole forest is on fire.

Do you remember the game in which you sit in a circle and a message is passed from one person to the next? The sentence is often changed as it works its way around the group, quietly being passed from one person to the next. As the message is passed along, bits and pieces of the original words get left out or changed. By the time the message has completed the circle, it may sound vastly different to the original intended sentence.

Gossiping is a lot like that game. As people pass on information about another person, they can often add their own slant on the story or exaggerate parts that sound better. By the time the hurtful gossip gets around, it can be far removed from the real truth and that's where extreme damage can be done.

I have a simple guidepost for working out if something is gossip or not: Ask yourself the following question before continuing to pass on information:

> *"Will this information build the other person up (make them feel great about themselves), or damage someone's self-image? Will I make that person feel bad?"*

It's simple, really. You will know, in your 'heart' whether the information is helpful or not. Use your intuition!

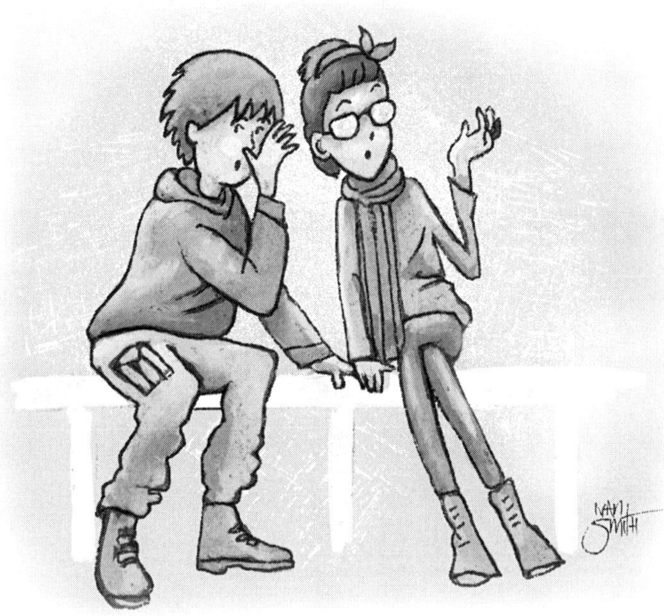

thoughts on bullying & gossiping

Watch the way you talk. Let nothing foul or dirty come out of your mouth. Say only what helps, each word a gift.

Ephesians 4:29
(The message)

'Gossip is only the lack of a worthy memory.'

Elbert Hubbard,
1856-1915

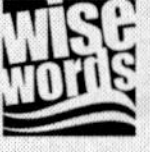

'Words kill, words give life; they're either poison or fruit—you choose.'

Proverbs 18:21
The Message

Gossips can't keep secrets, So never confide in blabbermouths.

Proverbs 20:18

'KIND WORDS ARE LIKE HONEY— SWEET TO THE SOUL AND HEALTHY FOR THE BODY.'

PROVERBS 16:24
NLT

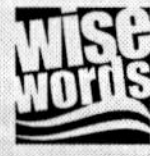

'A gadabout gossip can't be trusted with a secret, but someone of integrity won't violate a confidence.'

Proverbs 11:13
The Message

'Gossip needs no carriage.'

Russian proverb

'Live so that you wouldn't be ashamed to sell the family parrot to the town gossip.'

'The only time people dislike gossip is when you gossip about them.'

Will Rogers, 1879-1935

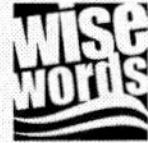

'For the Scriptures say, "If you want to enjoy life and see many happy days, keep your tongue from speaking evil and your lips from telling lies." '

1 Peter 3:10
NLT

Gossip is when you hear something you like about someone you don't.

Earl Wilson

'When of a gossiping circle it was asked, "What are they doing?"

The answer was: "Swapping lies".'

Richard Brinsley Sheridan, 1751- 1816

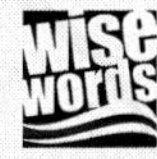

'Don't be bluffed into silence by the threats of bullies. There's nothing they can do to your soul, your core being. Save your fear for God, who holds your entire life — body and soul — in his hands.'

Matthew 10: 28
The Message

'Whoever gossips to you will gossip about you.'

Spanish proverb

...We are constantly bombarded

on a daily basis

with body images

that we cannot

live up to.

nine//

beyond perfection

navigating body image

no body's PERFECT!

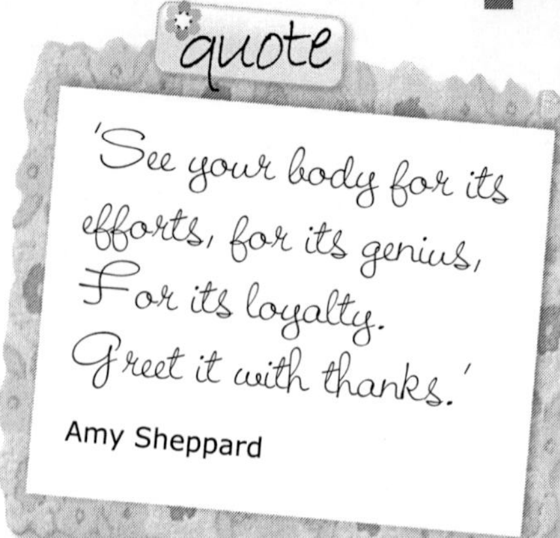

If you were to come away from reading this book with only **ONE** key message, it is this: **NO BODY IS PERFECT!** Every single girl has been created as UNIQUE, NEVER TO BE REPEATED, TOTALLY ORIGINAL, and ONE OF A KIND! This means that there is only ONE of you that will ever exist, and who you are is perfectly awesome.

Please re-read this last paragraph. It's important!

Body Image is a topic that many girls your age are concerned about and impacted by.

If you were to survey a thousand girls in your age group, the results would be close to one hundred percent of girls who experience mild concern, to overwhelming concern, at times, about their body.

When I was a teen girl, the only main influence we had on our changing bodies were the images we saw in magazines, advertisements, and on television programs. There was no social media, or the internet to bombard us daily with unrealistic images of body image perfection. It was much easier growing up in girl world back then.

quote

'How I feel about myself is more important than how I look. Feeling confident, being comfortable in your skin — that's what really makes you beautiful.'

Bobbi Brown

Whilst chatting with teen girls in a range of ages in preparation for writing this chapter, their collective sighs around the pressures of feeling like they need to live up to an unrealistic body image was overwhelming. As I listened to their deep connections as they shared how difficult it is to navigate the thousands of messages they receive each day through so many facets of the media, I was deeply concerned.

One teen shared:

'It's a lot of the Tik Tok and Instagram influencers that seem to affect me.

Seeing all these bikini models and perfect bodies – they all have these beautiful hour-glass figures.

The problem is, the more you scroll, the more these images appear in your social media feed.

It's difficult to escape it.'

Another teen girl, 13, added:

'One of my friends, Tayla, was involved in the modelling industry for some time. She stopped because of all the pressure she felt, comparing herself constantly to the other girls who she was modelling alongside. It took her down a difficult path, and she began wearing Hoodies and baggie tracksuit pants each day, so her body shape was disguised.'

If I could get ONE message to every single girl on the planet, it would be this:

BE YOU!

Everyone else is already taken

Who YOU are is ENOUGH!

There is NOONE else exactly the same as you in the entire universe!

One of my all-time favourite quotes is by Judy Garland, who famously played the part of Dorothy in the movie *The Wizard of Oz*:

quote

'Always be a first-rate version of yourself, Instead of a second-rate version of someone else.'

Judy Garland

I want this message to really sink into the depths of your soul.

YOU are amazing.

You are gorgeous – just as you are!

Over the past number of years, I have been involved occasionally in the media, and have appeared on various television programs as a commentator on teen issues.

One of the most telling comments once came from one of my students after they viewed my segment on replay.

'Mrs Witt! That doesn't really look like you on the screen.'

And the truth was – the image of me on the screen in front of them, propped beneath the bright lights of the television studio, was not realistic. Of course, it was a 'version' of me, however, it was a carefully prepared 'image' of me.

To further explain, when a guest, or television personality arrives at the studio to prepare for filming, they are ushered into the hair and makeup department. It is here that the transformation begins, with professional hair and makeup artists spending over an hour applying layers of makeup, concealer, and gloss to the lips, so that under the harsh glare of the studio lights, they will hopefully appear 'natural' on camera.

My hair would also be styled by a professional and sprayed so that it sat just right.

Studio lights are designed to be soft and flattering, so next time you see the faces of celebrities, or newsreaders on your TV screen, please run the dialogue through your mind that they have been prepared by a team of professionals to appear this way on your screen.

Many celebrities also engage stylists, whose job it is to locate outfits, shoes, and accessories and put these together to create a specific 'look.' Nothing you observe on your screens is by accident.

The key message I want you to understand is that a great deal of hard work goes on behind the scenes before a person generally makes an appearance on television, or any media appearance for that matter. And, yes, in case you are wondering, the males who appear on your television screens also receive the attention of the hair and makeup team.

becoming social media savvy

quote

'Social media is training us to compare our lives, instead of appreciating everything we are.'

Bill Murray

Every single day, we receive thousands of messages about how we should look, think, and act. If you are one of the millions of teenage girls around the country who has access to various social media platforms, you will receive many thousands more and I'll be perfectly honest, it can be really difficult for us adults to navigate, much less a young girl who is grappling with the changes associate with her growing and changing body.

Many celebrities and so-called social media 'influencers' have thousands, if not millions, of followers who devour every single image they upload on their carefully curated page.

You can most likely suggest some of the celebrities or well-known people you follow on social media. It is very easy to get stuck in the cycle of scrolling for hours just to see what others are up to in life- what they are wearing, where they are travelling, or what fun they are up to next. And it needn't just be well known people. We can get easily distracted by the images and stories our own friends and peers post on their socials.

We can so easily play the 'compare and despair' game.

But what are we really comparing ourselves to?

The truth is, almost every image we see on social media has not appeared by accident.

Influencers and celebrities may take hundreds of pictures of themselves, in various poses and outfits, before they carefully choose a particular filter, and upload the best version of themselves. Just imagine the time and effort that might go into just **ONE** image you glimpse on your social media feed!?

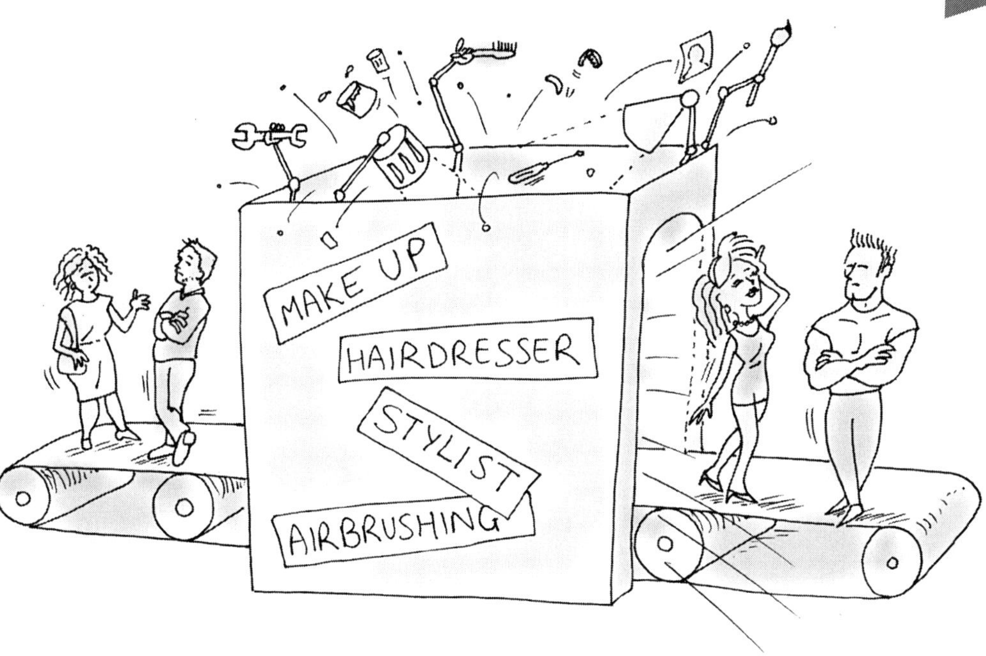

Dear Body,

You were never a problem.

There is nothing wrong with

your size or shape...

You are already good enough!

Love,

Me x

healthy role models to FOLLOW on your SOCIALS

quote

'You are a work of art. Divinely created and exquisitely designed.'

Shauna Ryan

Whilst there is an avalanche of social media identities that may cause us to feel inferior about our own perceived shortcomings about our bodies, there are plenty of amazing, strong gals you can follow on social media, who send clearer body positive messages on their feeds, and encourage others with their own inspiring stories.

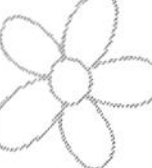

Amy Sheppard

One of my favourite gals to follow is Amy Sheppard @amysheppardpie

Amy is one third of the hugely successful Australian band, *Sheppard*.

She consciously posts positive messages on her social media accounts around being happy and LOVING your body. She regularly posts photos of herself in various locations, sometimes wearing her bathers WITHOUT use of filters or digital alterations.

She proudly shows her body in its natural state, never hiding any bumps or normal body fat that each of us have!

Amy recently posted this message, and I could not LOVE this MORE:

> *"Imagine if you could go back in time to visit your previous self. Would you go and look at that 10, 14, or 21- year- old in the eye and tell her that she was FAT, DISGUSTING, STUPID or UGLY? Chances are, you wouldn't.*
>
> *You'd probably give the poor girl a big hug and tell her that everything is ok and that she is beautiful and full of potential ... because she was!*
>
> *So now, go and look in the mirror and pretend that your future self is looking back on you as you are now. Look through the eyes of the 80- year -old person you will be one day; give the current you some appreciation, some adoration and tell her she is beautiful and is full of potential ... because she is."*
>
> *Amy Sheppard 2023*

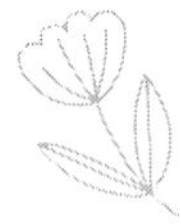

Turia Pitt

If you have never heard of the courageously strong woman, Turia Pitt @turiapitt I would wholeheartedly encourage you to read up on her incredible story.

In 2011, Turia was a mining engineer, living her dream in the beautiful Australian outback. Whilst competing in a 100-kilometre marathon, she was caught in a devastating grassfire and suffered extreme burns to sixty-five percent of her body. She made it out of the fire, barely alive, and battled over two-hundred medical procedures and undertaking two years of gruelling recovery to survive. Turia survived against overwhelming odds, and after her recovery, still has the visible signs of being so badly burnt. However, she is the image of true beauty!

Turia has completely rebuilt her life, got back into running, has had two beautiful boys, and inspires hundreds of thousands of people to not be caught up in how they look, but to embrace the miracle that is their body, and the incredible ways it can defy even the toughest odds, to recover. She inspires so many people today in her passion for running.

Turia has also written a brilliant book for teens called *Good Selfie – Tips and Tools for teens to nail life*.

You can read more about her story at www.turiapitt.com

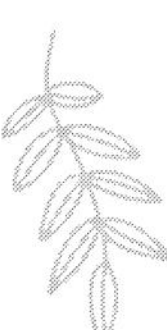

Shauna Ryan

Shauna Ryan @shaunashauna_ is another very cool Australian gal who is a digital content creator, speaker, writer, and model. She is incredibly inspiring because she fully embraces her body and curves, and regularly works with brands to model clothing for plus sized gals.

In Shauna's own words:

> *"I grew up never seeing women who looked like me, taking up space in cool rooms and events. I only saw plus-size women, hiding in corners, trying not to bring attention.*
>
> *So, I decided to become what I couldn't see.*
>
> *I became my own cheerleader.*
>
> *And I want to be yours too!"*

Shauna is such an inspiring woman because she chooses to embrace her curves, and actively chooses to LOVE her body for what it does for her, not conforming to what society would lead us to believe is the perfect body. The fact is your body IS perfect. Because it's yours!

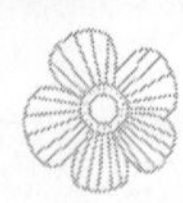

Taryn Brumfit

Taryn Brumfit @bodyimagemovement is another inspiring woman whose mission has become to educate and encourage girls and women to embrace their body in its entirety.

Taryn first caught media attention across the world, after she famously posted a 'before' and 'after' photo of herself after her pregnancy on social media, back in 2013. The image, and Taryn's message went viral (That means a LOT of people saw it and engaged with her messages!)

She went on to create films about body image, (check out *Embrace Kids* documentary), has written books and created programs to encourage others to embrace their bodies, and tackle the impossible standards of beauty often portrayed in the media. She was even awarded 'Australian of the Year' in 2023.

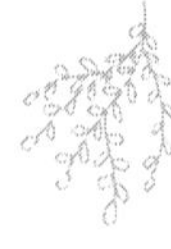

Samantha Gash

Samantha Gash @samanthagash rose to fame on Australian television screens when she appeared as a contestant on *Australian Survivor* in 2017, and on a later edition of the program in 2022. Sam is an accomplished lawyer, an endurance athlete and social impact leader. In her own words:

> *"If you want something you've never had – you must be willing to do something you've never done."*

This mantra has fuelled her remarkable journey of pushing mental and physical boundaries, creating lasting impact, and inspiring others to do the same.

Sam is small in stature, however, is one of the most inspiring and encouraging women I have the privilege of knowing. She encourages girls of every age to be physically healthy, and to push themselves to achieve their very best.

My list of positive female role models.

Make a conscious decision about who you CHOOSE to follow on social media

Think about this for just a moment...

YOU get to make the choice about **WHO** you choose to influence you.

You can make a conscious decision to **UNFOLLOW** social media accounts that do not make you feel good about yourself, and your body-image. There are plenty of inspiring and encouraging people that can positively influence your life and your social media feed.

Consider viewing it from this perspective – your mind and self-perception can be influenced positively or negatively based on your choices. Embracing unrealistic standards of body perfection constantly sends such messages to your brain.

Consider curating your social media by unfollowing accounts that don't contribute positively to your self-image and leave you feeling less than empowered and encouraged.

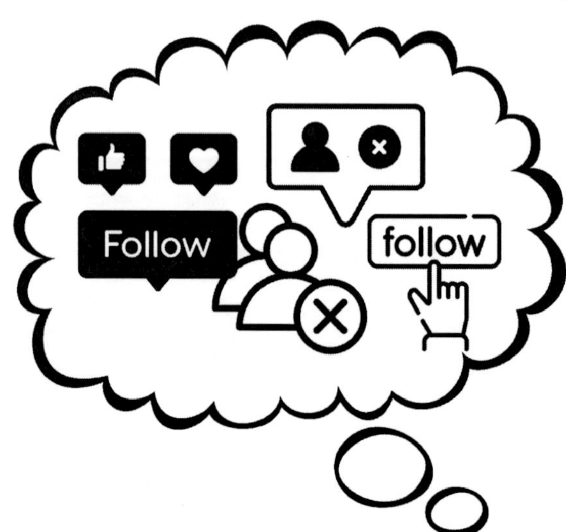

Take a Digital Detox

I want to encourage you to make it a regular habit to take a compete break from social media. (I know, it's a tough ask for many of you reading this!)

This not only gives your brain a great break to relax, imagine, create, and dream, but it will give YOU respite from the avalanche of images and messages that bombard you every time you open your device.

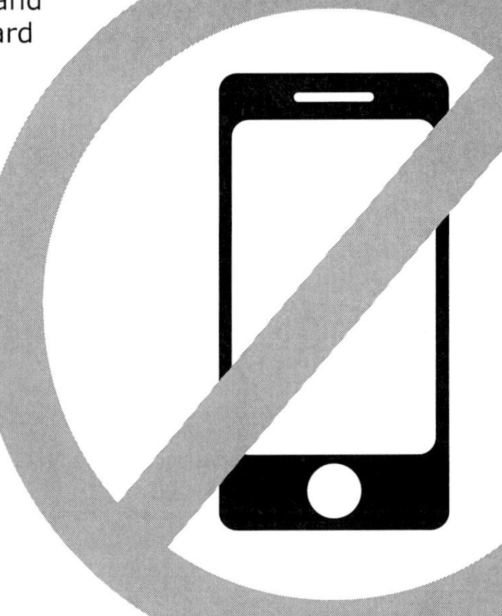

Consider going for an entire twenty-four hours of not opening your social media.

If you are already in the habit of scrolling daily, consider this a challenge.

Give yourself a break from the constant noise, chatter, and messages you receive when you open your social media feed – you deserve this, and so does your mind.

If you can take this challenge further, try going for two days, or even seven.

Your mind will thank you for it ☺.

Things you can do INSTEAD of going on social media

- **Read a Book:** Whether it's fiction, non-fiction, or a graphic novel, getting lost in a good book can be a great escape.
- **Start a Journal:** Writing can be therapeutic. It could be about daily life, dreams, or even creative stories.
- **Learn a New Skill:** Whether it's playing a musical instrument, painting, drawing, writing, sewing, cooking, pick up a new hobby.
- **Outdoor Activities:** Go for a hike, bike ride, or simply take a walk in the park. Fresh air does wonders.
- **Exercise:** Find a form of exercise you enjoy, whether it's pilates, dancing, or a sport. It's not just good for the body, but for the mind too.
- **Volunteer:** Give back to the community by volunteering at local organisations or events.
- **Start a Blog or YouTube Channel:** Share your thoughts, experiences, or creative endeavours with the world.
- **Learn a Language:** Use apps or online resources to pick up a new language. It's a valuable skill and can be a lot of fun.
- **Cook or Bake:** Experiment with new recipes and treat yourself to delicious homemade meals or snacks.
- **DIY Crafts:** Get creative with DIY projects. Whether it's making jewellery, crafting, or upcycling old items, it's a productive way to spend time.
- **Listen to Podcasts or Audiobooks:** Explore a variety of topics and learn something new while doing other activities.
- **Mindfulness and Meditation:** Practice mindfulness to help reduce stress.
- **Attend Workshops or Classes:** Many community groups offer courses on a wide range of subjects. It's a great way to expand your knowledge.
- **Play Board Games or Puzzles:** Have a games night with friends or family.
- **Photography:** Explore your surroundings and capture interesting moments with a camera or your smartphone.

Remember, the key is to find activities that bring joy and fulfillment!

helpful tips to build a positive body image

RECOGNISE UNREALISTIC BODY IMAGE STANDARDS

The first step towards developing a positive body image is acknowledging that the images portrayed on social media and in advertising are often carefully curated and manipulated. These images rarely reflect reality, as they have been edited to eliminate imperfections and highlight specific features. It's important to remember that no one looks flawless all the time, not even the people we see online.

CURATE YOUR FEED MINDFULLY

Take control of your social media feed. Follow accounts that promote body positivity, diversity, and self-acceptance. Surround yourself with content that celebrates all body types, ethnicities, and abilities. By seeing a variety of representations, you'll begin to internalise the idea that beauty comes in many forms.

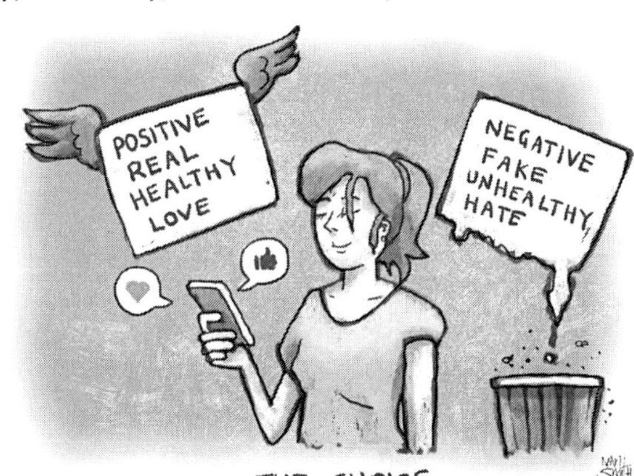

THE CHOICE...

LIMIT YOUR EXPOSURE

While social media can be a positive platform for self-expression and connection, it's also essential to set boundaries. Spending too much time comparing yourself to others online can lead to feelings of inadequacy. Allocate specific times for using social media and balance it with other activities that nourish your self-esteem.

UNDERSTAND THE PHOTOSHOP MYTH

Educate yourself about photo editing and how it can create unrealistic standards. Research before-and-after images to understand how even small changes in lighting, angles, and retouching can drastically alter appearances. This knowledge will help you see through the façade of flawlessness.

DIVERSE ROLE MODELS

Seek out role models who embrace their uniqueness and challenge societal norms. Identify people in your life or in the media who have achieved great things regardless of their body type. Their stories will serve as a reminder that your worth isn't determined by your appearance but by your character and achievements.

BUILD YOUR MEDIA LITERACY SKILLS

Developing media literacy skills is crucial in the digital age. Learn to critically analyse advertisements, articles, and videos. Ask questions like: What messages are they conveying? Are they promoting unrealistic ideals? How do they make you feel about yourself? By deconstructing media messages, you'll become a more empowered consumer.

SELF-COMPASSION AND SELF-TALK

Replace negative self-talk with self-compassion. Treat yourself with the same kindness and understanding you'd offer to a friend. When you catch yourself being self-critical, reframe those thoughts. Focus on your strengths, achievements, and the aspects of yourself that you appreciate.

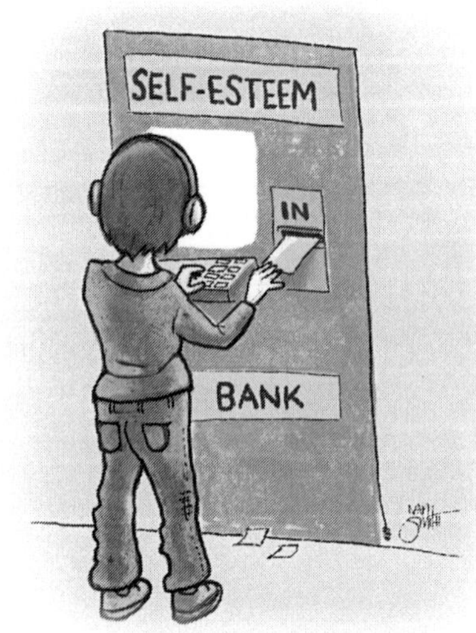

DEFINE BEAUTY ON YOUR TERMS

Beauty is not a one-size-fits-all concept. It's subjective and unique to every girl. Define beauty on your terms, embracing the qualities that make you special. Emphasise your talents, kindness, and the aspects of your personality that shine brighter than any physical attributes.

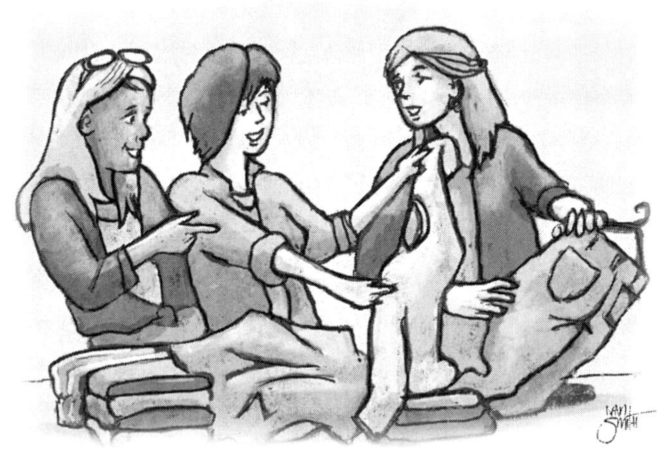

FOSTER REAL-LIFE CONNECTIONS

While social media can offer connection, real-life relationships are equally important. Surround yourself with friends who uplift and support you for who you are. Engaging in activities and hobbies that make you feel proud and accomplished can also boost your self-esteem.

PRACTISE SELF-CARE

Take care of your body and mind through healthy habits. Focus on nourishing foods, regular exercise, and sufficient sleep. Engage in activities that bring you joy and help you relax. When you prioritise self-care, you'll feel more in tune with your body's needs and appreciate it for all it does for you.

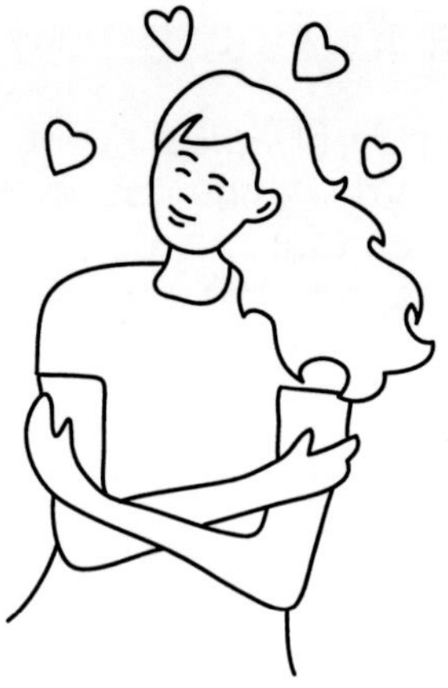

'Speak to your body
in a loving way.
It's the only one you've got.
It's your home and it
Deserves your respect.'

Iskra Lawrence

Thoughts from teen girls about Body Image...

Body image is something most of us struggle with; I definitely do.

As teenage girls there is a lot of pressure we feel to fit in, look pretty, and feel confident.

But that's not realistic. I know I really struggle with my body image; I mean I feel self-conscious just walking into school.

I know that I shouldn't have to worry about what people think of me, but it's hard not to. There are times when I feel very jealous of others and think that it's unfair that they can look like that. I shouldn't have to feel like this. I should be able to leave my house and feel confident in my body. This message isn't to make others feel like they should feel self-conscious, it's so that others know that its ok to feel like this, its normal. And if you struggle with body image you're not alone.

There are other girls out there that feel self-conscious of their body, so even when you feel like the world is against you, and you must fight this battle on your own, remember there are other girls out there fighting their own battles, thinking they are alone.

It's common to struggle with body image, but it shouldn't have to be. We shouldn't have to feel this way, and we shouldn't have all this pressure put on us. Even if people make you feel insecure, you can make sure that you don't do the same thing. Instead, you can give compliments to others. And just remember that you're never alone.

Grace, age 14

I have many friends who struggle with their body image, saying they are fat (when they are skinnier or weigh less than me.) I don't really worry too much because I love my body and it's the only body I'll ever have. I keep reminding my friends that their body is beautiful and perfect and the only people that call themselves fat are themselves. No one cares about what other people think but their own thoughts. I think girls and women should stop worrying if their body will fit a bikini or a bodysuit. I feel like they need to acknowledge their body for what it is. It isn't what's on the outside it's on the inside that counts.

Ella, age 14

Body image is something I have always struggled with, especially after the age of 11, mostly because of seeing other girls and always comparing myself with them. Or hearing people say things like "have you gained weight?", "are you really going to go out wearing that?" or "Wow, you eat a lot for your age".

I've been trying to love my body and fight all those thoughts telling me to not eat to the point of getting lightheaded and feeling sick, but it's easier said than done.

Aysa, age 14

Being a teenage girl is not easy. Especially with the
influence of social media.

All those girls with pretty faces, nice hair, and skinny
waists, makes me feel bad about myself. It's never good
enough for anyone. They always want you to have good
posture, be a nice person without being a pushover,
eating enough food but not too much that it makes you
look greedy, be skinny but not so skinny it makes you
look sick or unwell. But one thing you can do is believe
in yourself, look in the mirror and smile. Laugh ugly, eat
as much food as you want, and if those around you say:
" Oh you're eating so much " or " Are you really going to
wear that?" you can reply with: " No. I love myself, and
yes, I am going to eat all this food because I am hungry!"

Love yourself unconditionally,
YOU ARE AMAZING! ☺

Poppy, age 14

I often struggle with my body image.

Most people struggle with their body image.

Being a teen can be challenging and overwhelming
as you are always being forced to be shaped and
morphed into a perfect image for society. This
encourages us to eat more, eat less, get shaved
legs, hide our stretch marks, get smooth skin, and
a lot more.

I think we should all change the way we think
about our body image and start eating the way we
want, dressing the way we want, leaving our skin
the way we want, and just being ourselves.

Every girl should be treated equally as we are all
different and beautiful.

To be honest I am still overcoming this. However,
I now feel so much better as I know that I have
many people going through this with me.

Trianna, age,14

Being a teenage girl isn't easy. So many girls struggle with body image issues, including me. There is often so much pressure to look perfect, to be pretty, to fit in. I can't count the number of times I have looked in the mirror and wished the reflection looked different. Society and social media put so much pressure on teenage girls to look, act, and be perfect all the time, and it just isn't fair.

So many of us have such low self-esteem because of all the judgment from society about how we look and how we act. We don't deserve all the breakdowns and tears. I just wish that I could be confident in my body, and not always be worrying about what others think of me. There's always so much pressure to not eat too much, to have nice hair, to be skinny, to have a pretty face, to look pretty when you cry, but it's so unrealistic. Nobody can be perfect, and nobody should have to be perfect to fit in.

People need to learn to be happy with themselves and be confident in their own skin. Everybody is unique and special, and that's what we need to remember when people judge us. We need to learn to look in the mirror, and love what we see. We all deserve to be happy, and we all need to notice that we are beautiful in our own way, even if nobody else can see it. Always remember, you are not the only one who struggles with body image, and you are not alone! The most important thing is to love yourself!

Denali, age 14

Body image and how your body 'should look' are things that a lot of girls are taught about and exposed to from a very young age. Thinner, wider hips, smaller face, big eyes and so much more. Many girls aren't taught anything different, and it isn't healthy. Everywhere, different body types are advertised as 'perfect'. I know that for me personally, this has caused me to think that a lot of things about me that are healthy are, imperfect, and ugly. This hurts a lot of girls and can cause serious disorders and medical issues. I struggle with the way I look and eating enough because I can always find someone 'better' than me. But the perfect body type changes all the time and you shouldn't feel any less because you look different. Your body isn't fast fashion. It's beautiful and unique to you.

Mia, age 13

If you're insecure about your body, it's okay!

My advice is to guard your own body and don't let anyone, or a mirror ruin your self-esteem, it's up to you, YES YOU! You get to decide how you feel and what you do with your own body. 81% of the photos you see online are photoshopped and edited and that isn't okay. When you see a photoshopped photo, block and/or quickly scroll down so they won't pop up regularly on your page or feed.

Ashlee, age 14

Social media can make you think a lot about your body-image.

You can start to think about things like if people are talking about you and it just gets bad. You might not want to go out or socialise, but really it doesn't matter what you look like and what people think if you're happy within yourself. I don't have social media, so I don't look at that stuff like that.

Emily, age 14

I believe that body image is often perceived as a negative, however, it can also be positive, when the people around you or those you run into when scrolling through social media can have an impression and cause you to reflect on yourself. Whether it's the slim waist or the beauty standards or even the comments, these can have an influence on us and many other girls around the world. By surrounding yourself with positive people and the things you love, it can set the tone of respecting your own body image and loving yourself for who you were made to be. This has made me as a young teenage girl, love myself more rather than editing myself.

Irin, age 15

Body image is constantly being thrown in my face. It's something that I struggle with as I've faced many challenges with trying to love my body for the way it is. However, I've noticed how challenging it is to do that with everything else going on, whether that be what social media defines as a "good body" or what family members and individuals say about my body. I take note of how people's opinion on my body really gets to me negatively and try desperately to change my body just to fit their standards of what a perfect body looks like. As I've grown older though, I've chosen to block out all the negative comments people have to say about my body and understand that their definition of a perfect slim body is not realistic and never will be.

Adawt, age 15

Body image can be a difficult and sensitive topic. I personally think that social media is the biggest influence on why body image has become such a controversial topic because of companies, ads and stories that choose a selected group of people with similar body shapes and sizes to advertise through magazines, stores, social media, and more. This presents the idea of an "ideal body" which now I believe is the reason why teenagers have this imagery and standard of what a "good" body looks like.

Abby, age 16

I always thought, growing up, that I'd be confident in my body. How very wrong I was!

I find it so difficult not to compare myself to my peers.

For example, one of the girls at my school, 'Star' is literally the most perfect girl, with the brightest smile along with an hourglass figure.

I was involved in dance classes for six years, and always noticed other girls whom I saw as more beautiful, and with seemingly perfect bodies doing ballet and looking stunning in their dance costumes.

When I went into Year 7, I felt my world come crashing into pieces as issues with my poor body image came along at the same time I was dealing with some other issues. I even began restricting what I would eat in case I gained extra weight. This led me to becoming very, very unwell. Thankfully I received the help I needed, and I am well on the road to recovery.

For me personally, I think social media accounts like Tik Tok, and Instagram make me feel self-conscious of my body. Seeing all the bikini models and influencers with beautiful bodies, all seeming so confident, is difficult for me to navigate and not compare myself.

I tend to feel better about my body after I play a game of football because when I play sport, it is much less about what your body looks like, but what it can do. It teaches me that my body is way more capable than what I believe it is.

We are still only kids, and it may seem silly, but the right amount of food for your body energises you. If you don't get enough nutrition, your body will suffer. When I think of how unwell I became, it all links back to not feeling good about my body and I now feel terrible about what I put it through. I now share my story with others so they will understand how bad it can be to not care for your body and suffer the consequences of this.

Lexie, age 13

Around this time last year, I was bullied for my body hair.

Since then, I have never felt happy going to pool and beaches, hearing girls complain about their legs being hairy after shaving two days ago, can be really difficult to hear because I have to wait up to three to six weeks for my legs to be smooth because I get my legs waxed.

For all you girls who get your legs waxed, please listen to me when I say this – please don't feel ashamed of this! I know that it can suck sometimes, but I now have learnt to live with it. It took me so long to accept it and feel happy with my body hair and ignore all of things she was saying about me. The first three months after I was bullied, I wasn't myself – and I wasn't eating much either.

Just because you get your legs waxed, you shouldn't be ashamed of it. Be yourself. And if you feel insecure about it, just remember that everyone has it, and you are beautiful no matter what!

Emmerson, aged 14

Since Grade one, people have made fun of my body. I've never really been what you'd call a skinny girl, which I've learnt to be okay with. But all through primary school I was bullied for my body, it put me down so much. The thing I hated the most was the bullies were calling me names every single day. And then, knowing that it hurt me so much, they just did it more.

After four years at my primary school, I moved to a different school. Unfortunately, the bullying happened there too, but it was worse! In grade six, I started to play netball. I was so looking forward to playing however, even at training, girls made fun of my weight, causing me to cry during most training sessions.

In year seven, I moved to another school for high school. I was really worried that I was going to be bullied there too, however I was fortunately wrong.

Everyone was so welcoming, friendly and I was so happy.

The friends I made helped me feel happy and confident in myself. I am fourteen now.

Girls my age don't need to feel embarrassed about their body.

It's YOUR body and YOUR rules.

Embrace your beauty because life is too short not to because we are all beautiful.

Greta, aged 14

As you finish reading this chapter about body image, I would encourage you to re-read the messages and stories within a second time and revisit it many times over.

Consider using a highlighter to emphasise points or quotes that resonate with you.

I would also suggest using some post it notes to earmark pages that you would like to read over and over, until the ideas sink in.

It can take time to fully digest the important messages about learning to love and appreciate the one body that you have been given.

And just in case you needed to be reminded yet again...

You are totally amazing.

Just the way you are!

quote

'I definitely have body issues, but everybody does. When you come to the realisation that everybody does that – even the people that I consider flawless – then you can start to live with the way you are.'

Taylor Swift

the world is your mirror

Have a look in a mirror. What do you see?

Is the person in the mirror always frowning, despairing?

Is the 'default' (or average) look a down one, a picture of negative self-esteem rather than positive?

Well that is in fact, what others will see, if you choose to reflect it. You reflect to others who you are and how you want to be treated. Try walking around with a smile and practise having a healthy self-esteem, even if you don't really feel it's true. The amazing thing is that people will begin to respond to your attitude. They really will!

Quite often, the esteem you give yourself is much lower that what others think of you. You may say, 'I'm a pretty boring, unpopular person'. If you actually believe that and reflect it to others, you'll probably end up being that sort of a person. But if you choose to reflect an image of being happy and wanting to spend time with others, it will happen.

Just watch!!

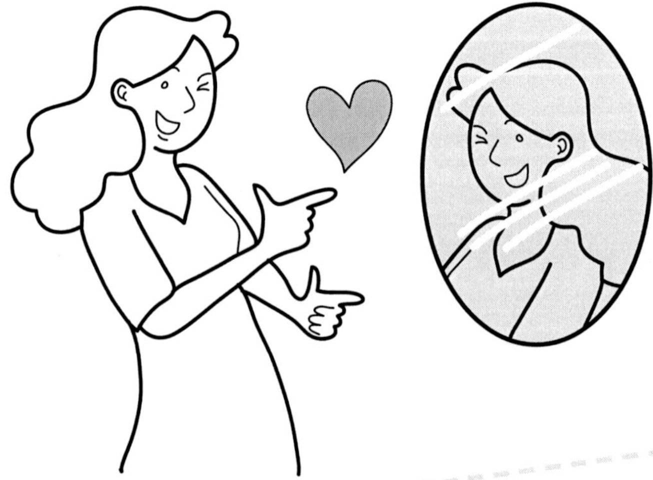

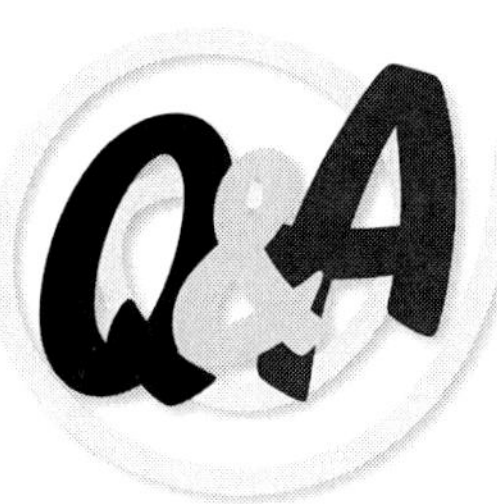

If you are comfortable with how you look, others will follow the feelings you have about yourself because you will give off a radiance and confidence that will attract others to you. Mostly, you need to feel comfortable with yourself, so try not to worry too much about the clothes you wear and how your hair should be. Your friends and family will accept you for the fantastic and amazing person you are.

Why do some girls care so much about their appearance?

Taking care with your appearance is generally a normal part of growing up, but try not to let it control you! When feeling a bit emotional or tired, we can often feel a bit *yuck* about ourselves. Doing your hair nicely and wearing a cool outfit can often give you a bit of a lift. Some girls, however, do become overly obsessed with how they look and dress. Not only does this become exhausting for the girl concerned, but just think about the extra pressure that it adds to other girls. Obsessing with hair, makeup and clothing is actually a massive time waster. Be more concerned with what's going on with the inside of you. After all, that's where your true beauty radiates from!

When I look in the mirror, all I can see is 'fat' with a capital 'F'!

News Flash! This can actually happen to everyone! Even the most gorgeous celebrities and super models have 'fat' days — they look in the mirror and are shocked by the image staring back. Many, many, many girls and women see themselves as fat at various times. Try not to look in the mirror too much. Those panels of glass often lie anyway!

The worst place to look at yourself in the mirror, incidentally, is the fitting room of a department store! Bad idea! Those big fluorescent lights emphasise every single lump and bump that you have on your body and give you a totally unrealistic view of how you really do look under natural light.

Your true beauty is in the whole package — how you act towards others, how you appreciate and love yourself and the worth you give to yourself!

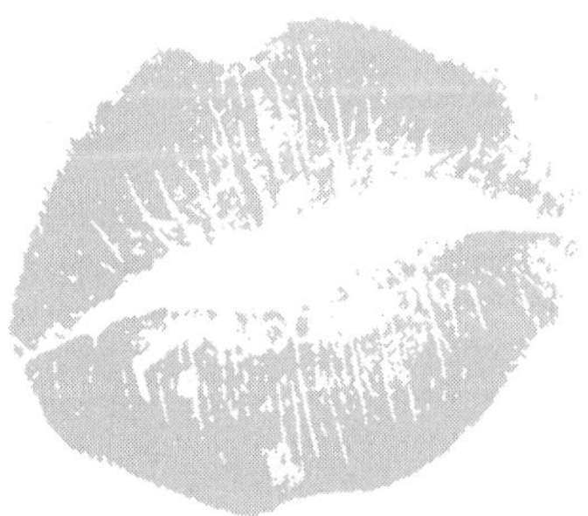

Your true beauty is in the whole package — how you act towards others, how you appreciate and love yourself and the worth you give to yourself!

ten//

What's the deal with boys?

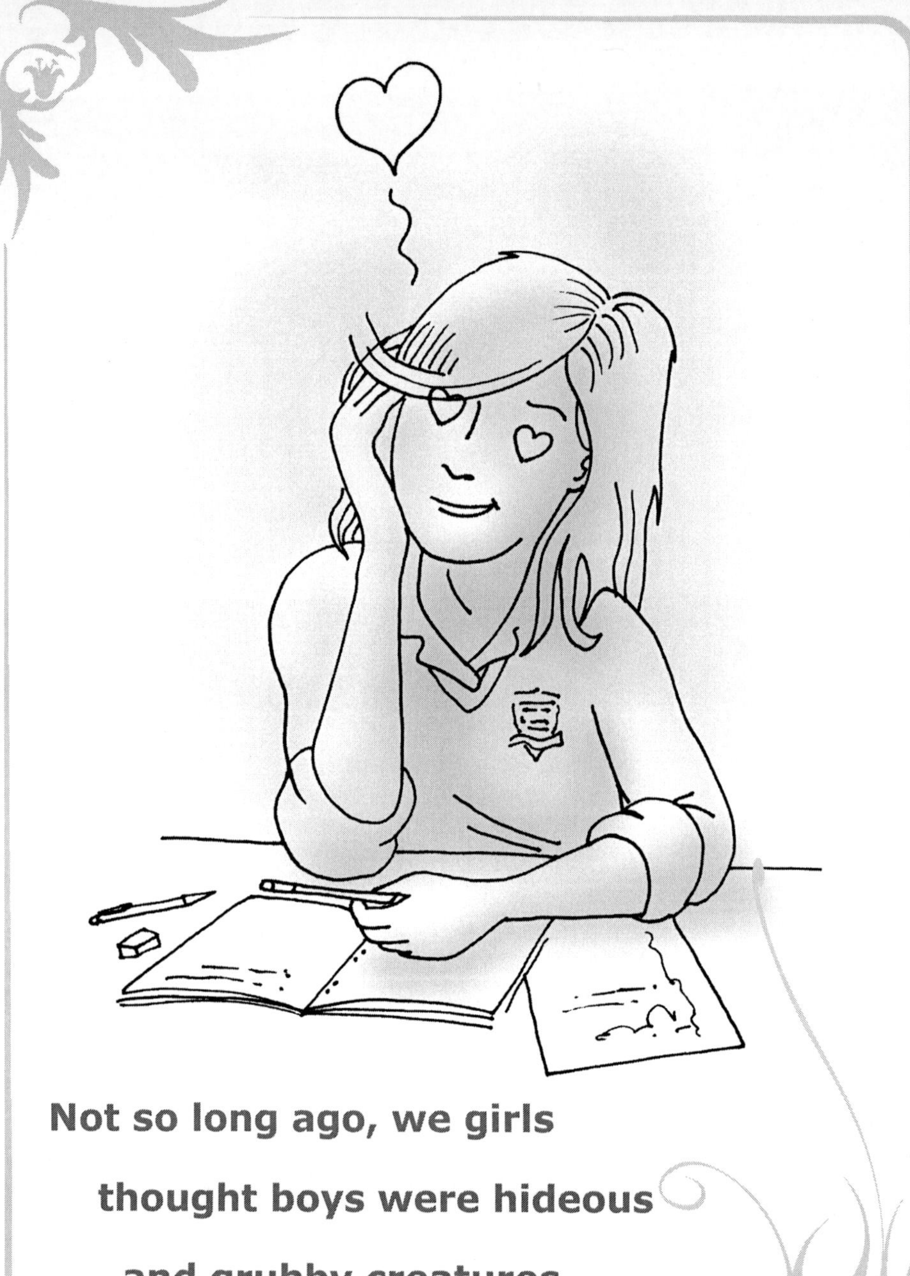

Not so long ago, we girls thought boys were hideous and grubby creatures...

boys, boys, bOYS!

Have you ever sat in class and just couldn't concentrate on anything at all other than the cute guy sitting on the other side of the room?

Your mind wanders. You imagine what it would be like to actually kiss him. You picture your wedding day, all your friends with you to celebrate your wonderful union; the cute house that you'll set up together and your gorgeous twin girls who will complete your new family—

'Jessica, what's the answer?'

'What's the answer? I don't even know the question!'

Your mind switches back and you realise that you're not on a picnic with your gorgeous husband and twin daughters, but you are in fact in your Year 8 Maths class and Mr Morris is standing in front of your desk, *Maths Essential Unit One* open to page 92!

'Sorry Mr Morris,' you reply.

'Well maybe next time you'll pay attention!' Mr Morris replies, angrily.

When our minds click into 'boy mode' it can seem that this stage of our teen years is just completely consumed by the opposite sex. Not so long ago, we girls thought boys were hideous and grubby little creatures who only liked playing footy and getting dirty. Now, all of a sudden it seems, boys appear to be a little sensitive, cute and the object of our new affections. Why is this?

>>>

Basically, our hormones have switched into a new gear, and at this point, boys seem a little different than they once were. It is quite a common occurrence for girls to seem totally 'boy–focussed' or 'boy crazy'. We daydream about guys we like and can seem totally obsessed with one boy one minute, and then wonder what we ever liked about him the very next. This is all perfectly normal! Try to enjoy this time but remember that the first boy that you have a crush on is most likely not going to be the boy you'll end up with.

We daydream about guys we like and can seem totally obsessed with one boy one minute, and then wonder what we ever liked about him the very next.

why do I have to like GUYS so much?

Good question! Let's face it, it would be a lot easier navigating those nasty teenage years without the issues of the opposite sex going hand-in-hand with growing up. Some girls seem to fly through their teenage years without really bothering too much about guys, but they are perhaps in the minority.

Most girls will wake up at some point and suddenly look at a guy at school in a whole new light. It's those lousy hormones again! Yes, they're the culprit. They make us lose our focus in Drama class, where we can only stare at the same guy and our attention is anywhere but what the teacher is saying. Suddenly, everything the boy says is humorous and that ugly way he styles his hair is, all of a sudden, pretty cute.

At that point, it really ***does*** matter to you what you wear to school, because if you pay so much attention to a guy, imagine how much attention they are paying to you. (In actual fact, many adolescent boys are not particularly cluey when it comes to girls liking them and many are not too interested in girls). Remember, guys tend to go though maturity at a later stage than girls.

It is common for girls to do some strange things when infatuated with a boy. Pursuits such as finding out where they live, and looking up the street are pretty normal things (I'm not quite sure if collecting a guy's lunch wrappers everyday and keeping them in a container is normal, but it has happened!).

You may find yourself talking to their mates (*or asking their friend to ask his friend what he thinks of you!*) and it's all perfectly normal.

A teenage girl asked me recently, 'Is it normal for me to *always* have to like a boy, at any given time?' My reply was, 'Yes, it is all perfectly normal. In fact you'll probably like a whole series of different boys at many different stages whilst you're a teenager, and beyond. It's just another phase of growing up and becoming a young woman.'

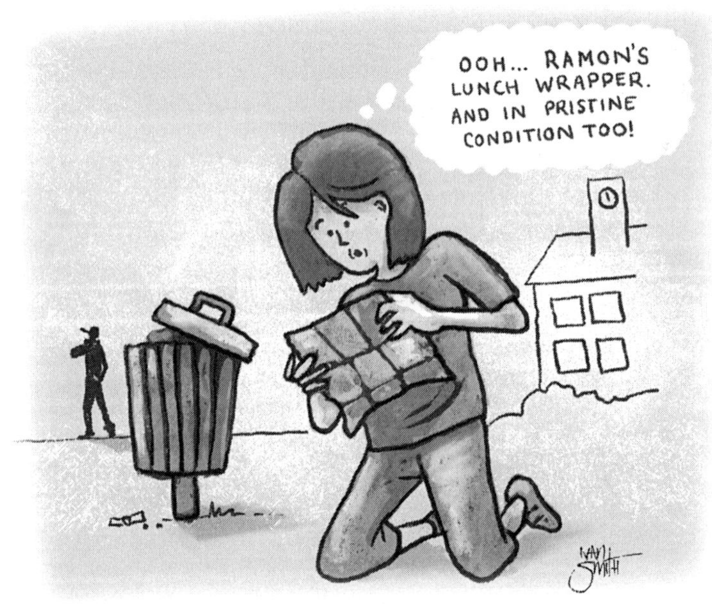

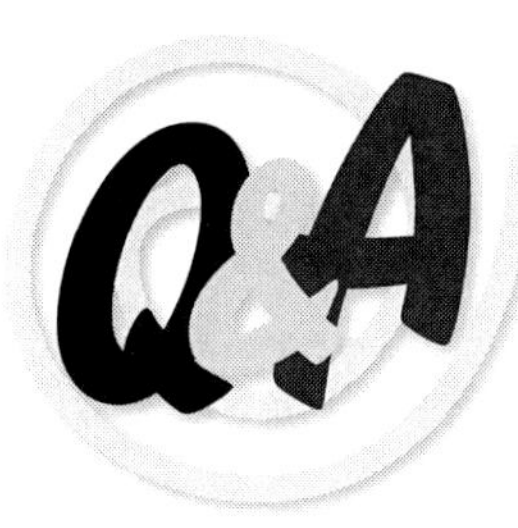

I really like this boy, but I'm too shy to talk to him. I think about him all the time, and when I do talk to him, I go all red and stutter.

Is it normal to like a guy this much?

During your teenage years, it is definitely normal to become just a little obsessed with boys. You can blame this again on those dreaded hormones! It is also pretty safe to assume that you'll change which boy you like, quite often.

Because our hormones are circulating, boys can become one of our main focus points. Where once you wouldn't look twice at a boy in that way, you soon find that you can think of nothing else. It can feel like your body and mind has been totally taken over by your hormones.

Why do boys sometimes treat us really bad when they really like us a lot?

Just like you sometimes feel awkward and unsure how to act around boys, guys feel exactly the same around girls a lot of the time. Where they weren't even remotely interested in girls previously, they soon can't stop thinking about them. But at this point, it becomes a little awkward. 'How do I act?' he asks himself. 'What if she realises that I like her?'

When boys tease you or play around with you, it's usually because they are unsure of what to say, and how to act around girls. One important point worth noting is that it is ***never okay*** for a guy to talk to you in a disgusting or sexually suggestive way. It is also ***never okay*** for a boy to physically hurt a girl! This is called abuse and it is against the law.

teach guys how to treat you!

Boys are also navigating adolescence and are learning how to relate to girls on a whole different level. Whereas they were accustomed to simply mucking around in the playground with girls, or playing chasey, they soon notice that all is not the same in the girl world. Some boys might start to pick on girls because they are trying to work out how to best relate to them.

This is where you come in! Boys will be guided and educated by the behaviour you allow when they are around you. You may find that boys like to make jokes or say cruel things about your changing body. It's really important that you send a clear message that it is ***not okay*** to make jokes about your body (or anyone else's).

Boys will be guided by the behaviour you allow them to get away with when they are around you.

You may notice that boys suddenly become a little more aware that girls are developing breasts and their body is changing. They need to be very mindful of treating you with respect. If you send a clear message by ignoring boys who make unwanted comments, or walk away from them, you soon send a very clear message that you will not settle with being treated any less than you deserve. **If you have the chance, ask a boy if he would be happy with a guy talking to his mother or sister in that way.** He should soon get the message.

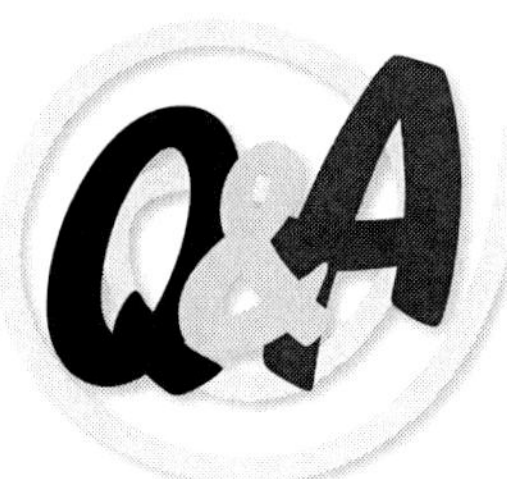

Why do some boys seem so immature?

That may be because some are!

It is commonly known that boys tend to experience puberty a bit later than girls do. You may be almost fully developed, physically, as a teenager, yet boys of a similar age are still walking around with scrawny bodies and squeaky voices. Eventually though, everyone catches up, but it's quite normal for boys to seem a bit immature – it's all a typical part of adolescence.

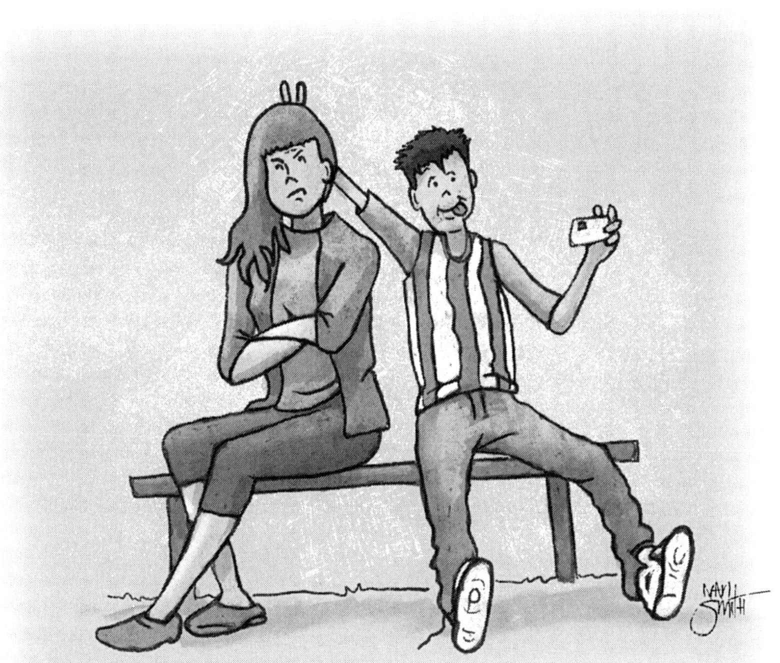

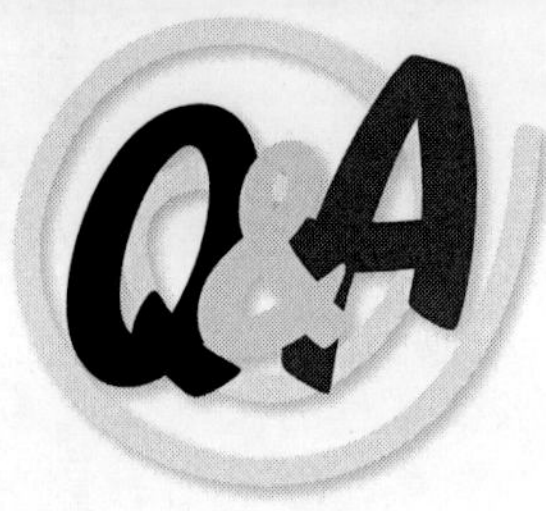

How do I tell a boy that I like him?

The quite obvious answer to this one is you tell him.

This is, however, quite often easier said than done, particularly when you're right in the midst of adolescence. It's always important to be yourself and not worry too much about boyfriends and taking a relationship too seriously.

Enjoy your teenage years and try not to let relationships with boys get in the way of the gift that is your time of growth.

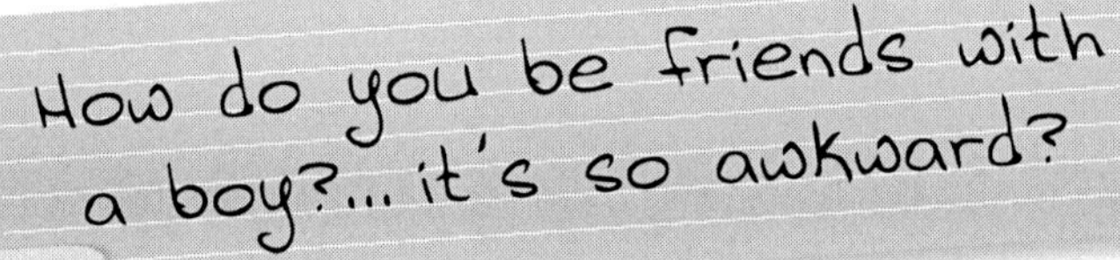

Once girls hit puberty, there often comes a point where boys suddenly look different to you. Where once you barely took notice of boys, suddenly you begin to see them in a totally different light. You start to take note of how you dress and act in front of a boy's company.

Then there always comes the question: 'How do you remain friends with a boy, without all that girl/boy pressure and hassle?'

There are times when it can feel a bit awkward, but the best advice is to just be yourself. By this I mean, don't try to be anyone other than who you truly are. Not only is it possible to be friends with boys, it's actually a very healthy thing! Don't rush into anything more than this. Being friends with boys is the best way to learn how to develop honest relationships with them without hassles. It is possible, and preferable, to learn to relate with and understand boys in a non-threatening environment.

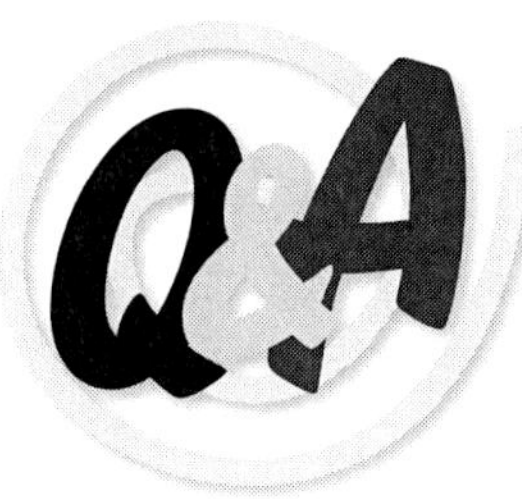

How do you break up with a guy, and remain friends?

Being a girl and going through adolescence is difficult enough, without all the pressure of boys and attaching yourself to one guy in particular.

In my humble opinion, it's better to be friends with boys during your early teen years, rather than confining your affections to one boy in particular. There is plenty of time down the track for boyfriends, however I'm sure there will be times when you also want to officially 'go out' with a boy. It makes us feel valued and wanted, but it's important that you learn to accept yourself and value yourself for who you are, not for what a boy thinks of you.

Breaking up with anyone is difficult because you are dealing with someone else's feelings — coping with a sense of rejection — emotions that are never pleasant.

Try to remember this: It's always better to break up with someone in person. Breaking up through a third party (eg: getting your best friend to pass on the message) is just poor taste. At least have respect and care to say it face-to-face. Text or private message breakups are also foolish and likely to both offend and confuse. Just remember that the person will often feel rejected no matter what you say, so it's important to reassure them of their value and worth.

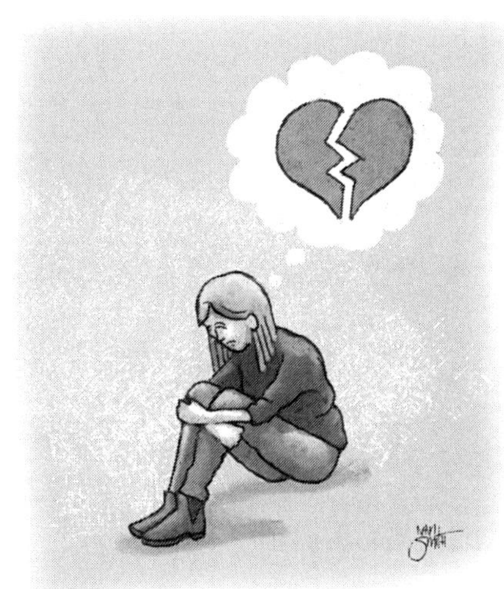

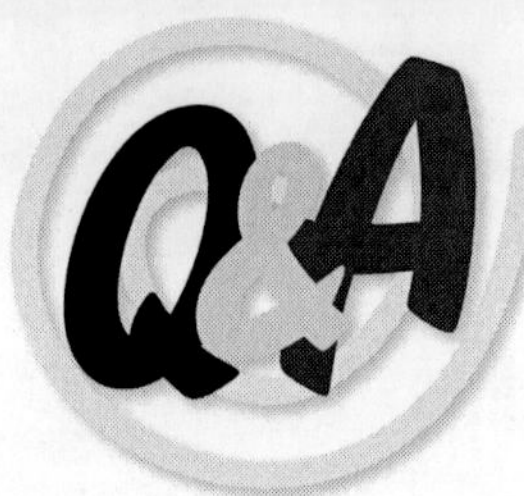

Why do some guys act like such jerks?

When experiencing these tricky years of adolescence, both girls and guys can, at times, act silly or out of character. Be it hormones or confusing body image, you are all still trying to work out who you are and where you fit in.

Sometimes, boys can just say and do silly things because they are trying to work out how to best relate to girls on a totally new level. Whereas 'BP' (before puberty) girls were just pals and meant nothing, they become a lot more interesting and attractive.

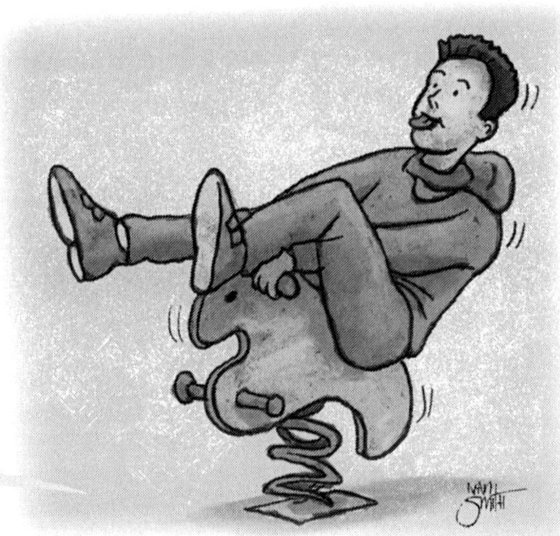

Bottoms, boobs and legs – why do guys seem so obsessed?

Guys are generally attracted to these parts of a girl's anatomy. It's just a part of their genetic makeup (the way they were designed). Because boys begin seeing girls in a whole new light, they are naturally going to find those parts of a girl more appealing.

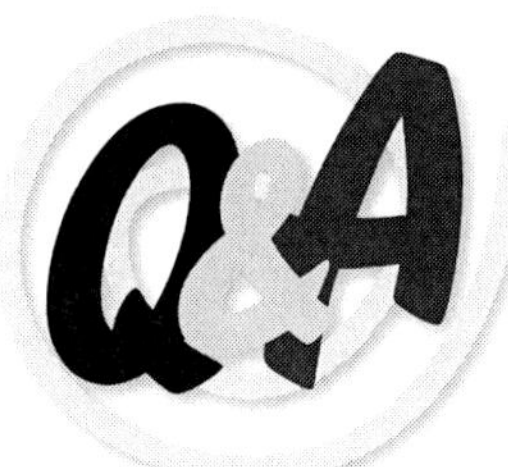

Why do guys put girls down all the time, saying they're just joking?

If a guy puts down a girl by saying something rude or degrading, first of all, it is not okay and you should ***never accept*** that type of behaviour! Put-downs are basically a form of bullying, and if they continue after you have told a boy to stop, you need to let a trusted adult, parent or teacher know about the problem. Often guys use put-downs as a 'cover' for how they really feel because they are dealing with their own feelings of worth.

Rather than simply saying they like you, boys can make silly teasing remarks that they know will get a reaction from you. Usually, they don't really mean to be nasty, but they are trying to work out in their own minds how to relate to girls on a new level. If a guy annoys you with silly remarks or inappropriate behaviour, make sure you tell them quite clearly that it is not okay! In my experience, most boys, once they have been told how a girl has reacted, feel pretty bad. It's a whole new learning experience for them too.

Should I have a boyfriend at the age of 13?

Having a boyfriend is a fairly big step at any age.

My advice here is to try and stay friends with a range of boys. Learn how to relate to guys as friends before you step into the new realm of dating and boyfriends. Wait until you're much older — say 16+, before you start dating. At age 13, you're not really likely to find your life partner, nor should you be looking, and that's really what dating is all about. There is too much to enjoy and experience at age 13 without all the hassles of boyfriends. There will be plenty of time for that later, and believe me, that time will come around quicker than you can blink!

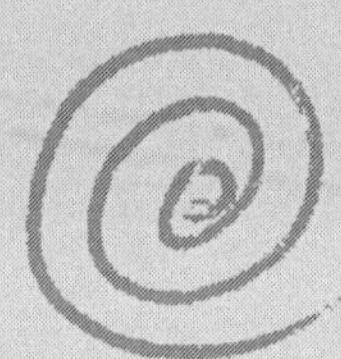

"I am always doing the best I can,
If I could do better,
I surely would.
And when I can, I surely will."

Robyn Posin

"Take chances, make mistakes.
That's how you grow.
Pain nourishes your courage.
You have to fail in order
to practise being braver."

Mary Tyler Moore
American actress

eleven//

caring for your mental health

caring for your mental health

> *"Slow breathing is like an anchor in the midst of an emotional storm: the anchor won't make the storm go away, but it will hold you steady until it passes."*
>
> *Russ Harris*

I had a fantastic and reliable car a few years ago. It ran like a dream and never let me down, until one day it died. It had been a couple of stressful years (I'm talking about you COVID!) and, well, I missed a couple of important services on my car.

Because I had failed to maintain my car properly, I had not noticed that the oil was low and before I knew it, my car engine had run out of oil. This resulted in what the mechanic called 'catastrophic engine failure.' It was a very tough, not to mention expensive, lesson to learn.

Maintaining our mental health is not unlike caring for a car – we must pay attention to it and ensure we put in the necessary measures to maintain our wellbeing.

Approximately one in five young people experience mental health concerns, so if you are experiencing anxiety, depression or struggling in any way, you are not alone.

As a young person, you may experience a wide range of emotions and feelings as you navigate the challenges of growing up. From academic pressure to social anxiety, it's easy to feel overwhelmed and stressed out.

However, taking care of your mental health is just as important as taking care of your physical health. Here are some tips on how to prioritise your mental health:

Connect with others

CONNECTING WITH OTHERS can help you feel less alone and more supported. Talk to your friends, family members, or a trusted adult about how you're feeling. If you don't feel comfortable talking to someone you know, consider seeking professional help. A therapist or counsellor can provide a safe space for you to talk about your thoughts and feelings. There are also some really helpful phone numbers and website supports listed at the end of this book, should you want to chat to someone anonymously about how you are feeling.

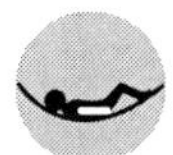

Practice self-care

SELF-CARE is all about taking care of yourself physically, emotionally, and mentally. Make sure you're getting enough sleep, eating healthy foods, and exercising regularly. Take breaks when you need them, and do activities that you enjoy, such as reading, listening to music, or spending time outside. Practicing self-care can help you feel more balanced and energised.

Manage stress

STRESS is a natural part of life, but too much stress can be harmful to your mental health. Identify your sources of stress and try to manage them. This might involve prioritising your tasks, breaking them down into smaller, more manageable steps, and setting realistic goals. Additionally, relaxation techniques such as deep breathing, listening to calming music, going for regular walks and getting out in nature, can help you calm down and reduce stress.

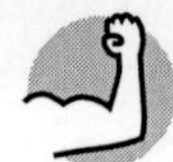

Build resilience

RESILIENCE – Building resilience can help you handle stress and adversity more effectively. To build resilience, try to focus on the things you can control, such as your thoughts and actions. Practice positive self-talk and try to reframe negative thoughts. Also, remember to take care of your physical health, as this can have an impact on your mental well-being. See the chapter about building your resilience earlier in this book.

Seek help when needed

If you're struggling with your mental health, it's important to **SEEK HELP**. This might involve talking to a trusted adult, such as a parent, teacher, or counsellor. Additionally, you can contact a mental health professional, such as a therapist or psychologist. There are also resources available, such as phone numbers, that you can use if you're feeling overwhelmed or in crisis. (*Please see the resources at the back of this book.*)

Taking care of your mental health is important at any age, but it's especially important during the teenage years when you're going through changes and challenges.

Remember to prioritise your mental health by connecting with others, practicing self-care, managing stress, building resilience, and seeking help when needed.

when you're feeling down

quote

"The struggle you're in today is developing the strength you need for tomorrow. Don't give up."

Robert Tew

If you are feeling down for any length of time (e.g., two weeks), it is important that you seek help. Being a teen can be tough at the best of times, and it is quite common to feel overwhelmed sometimes and be unable to cope. These feelings, however, should not last more than a couple of days. If you consistently feel sad and hopeless about your situation, it is important that you ask for help.

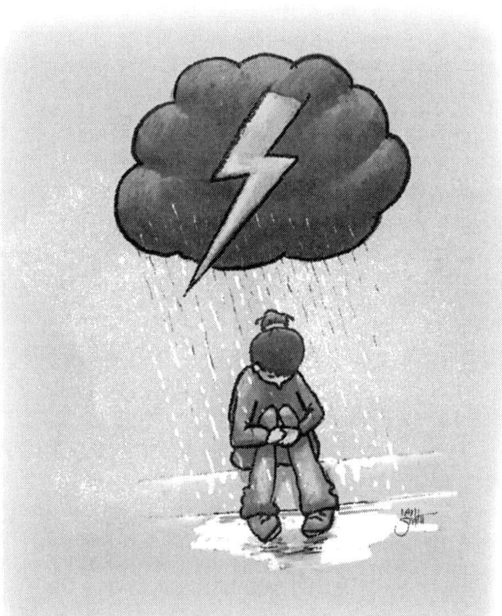

Talk to your parents, teacher, friend, school counsellor or coordinator, sister, brother, aunty, or church/youth group leader. Tell them honestly how you are feeling. If you feel that this is too much for you to cope with, please call one of the numbers at the back of this book. Trained people can also give you confidential advice and assistance.

SIGNS OF DEPRESSION

- *Feeling sad, hopeless.*
- *Crying often for no apparent reason.*
- *Extreme weight loss or weight gain.*
- *Lack of motivation and feeling like you cannot be bothered.*
- *Loss of interest in activities.*
- *Feeling tired and exhausted all the time.*
- *Feeling worried and anxious often.*
- *Sleeping too much or feeling like you need to sleep all the time.*
- *Turning to drugs or alcohol to cope with life.*

If you are feeling down for any length of time (e.g., two weeks), it is important that you seek help. Being a teen can be tough at the best of times, and it is quite common to feel overwhelmed sometimes and be unable to cope. These feelings, however, should not last more than a couple of days. If you consistently feel sad and hopeless about your situation, it is important that you ask for help.

Talk to your parents, teacher, friend, school counsellor or coordinator, sister, brother, aunty, or church/youth group leader. Tell them honestly how you are feeling. If you feel that this is too much for you to cope with, please call one of the numbers at the back of this book. Trained people can also give you confidential advice and assistance.

If you experience two or three of these symptoms for more than a week or two, please seek help from a trusted adult. There is so much support for you and you never ever have to be on this journey alone. You can also find some helpful websites and phone numbers to call at the back of this book.

MOOD BOOSTERS

- *Sleep*
- *Make a date with a friend and just vent*
- *Put on your runners and just walk*
- *Disconnect from social media for a period of time (delete the apps off your phone)*
- *Have a bubble bath and light some candles*
- *Take yourself on a dinner date for one*
- *Do something that brings you joy*
- *Begin a new craft or hobby*
- *Clean out your wardrobe/shoes and donate things you no longer wear to charity*
- *Bake some yummy food*
- *Have your hair professionally washed and cut*
- *Drive to the beach (or have a friend drive you) and spend the day reading magazines or a good book*
- *Walk through a forest*
- *Write*
- *Make a list of the things that are overwhelming you*
- *Paint*
- *Book to see a counsellor to talk things through*
- *Take yourself to the movies*
- *Wear pyjamas and watch movies all day*
- *Hike in a national park*
- *Listen to music*
- *Journal*
- *Forgive yourself*

THERE WILL BE SOME DAYS
YOU'LL FEEL LIKE GIVING UP –
THOSE TIMES THAT YOU DON'T THINK
YOU HAVE THE STRENGTH TO GO ON.

AND WITHIN EACH SECOND
THAT DOES PASS YOU BY RESIDES
GLIMMERING REMINDERS OF THE
MOST IMPORTANT PROMISE WHICH
MUST BE KEPT TO FUTURE YOU:
ONE THAT ENSURES YOU
MAKE IT THROUGH

defying Dread

Taming stress and anxious feelings

Have you ever walked down a flight of stairs and almost missed the last step? Or maybe you've woken in the middle of the night and remembered that you forgot to complete an important assignment due first thing in the morning? That instant feeling when your heart begins to race, and you feel like your mind is whirring? This is what anxiety can feel like, and it can happen to absolutely anyone; friends, your parents, teachers, doctors, actors – anyone at all. It doesn't discriminate.

If you ever feel the effects of anxiety, I want you to know that you are **NOT ALONE**.

In fact, I personally know many people that experience anxious feelings on a regular basis, and guess what?
I do too!

What causes anxiety?

When you can understand why we feel the effects of anxiety, it makes a LOT of sense.

It all stems from your **AMAZING BRAIN**.

Our brains have been designed to keep us safe.

Many years ago- in prehistoric times, our brain was very helpful at protecting us from very real threats of attacks by vicious animals and other groups of people.

When a threat was detected, a part of the brain called the **AMYGDALA**, leapt into action and released a powerful chemical called **CORTISOL**. This chemical causes a bodily response to protect the person and give them an extra boost to fight or run fast away from danger. This causes blood to rush to your most vital organ, your heart, to make sure it is pumping hard so you can run FAST or have extra strength to fight.

When we feel anxious, our heart might feel like it's racing.

Now if you are under real threat (such as about to be attacked by a gigantic gorilla) then your brain is doing exactly what it's been designed to do – protect you.

BUT!

Your very amazing brain cannot tell the difference between an **ACTUAL** threat (something that might cause you physical harm), and a **PERCEIVED** threat (something that may be concerning you but not a danger.)

If you aren't required to fight or run from that dangerous gorilla, there's no need for all that extra protective fuel that your brain has just released to give you strength. This can make you feel pretty yuck!

Here are some of the physical things that your body does when your brain sends out it's warning signal that your life might be at risk:

Brain – also controls your emotions, and you may feel a little teary.

Digestive system – goes into shut down mode to preserve energy whilst you run away or fight.

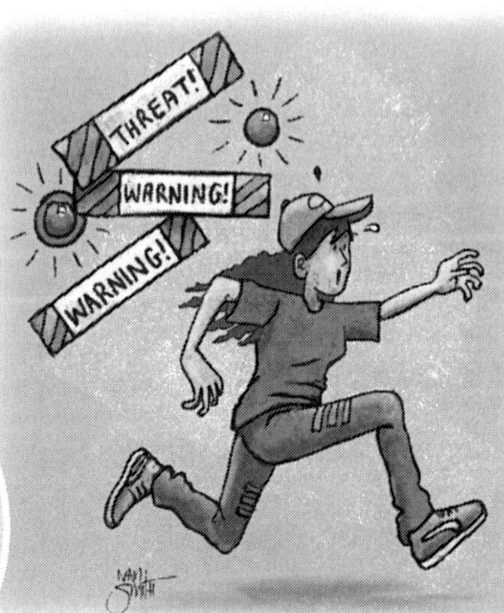

Legs – extra fuel sent to your legs in case they need to run. They may feel wobbly.

Sweat – your body tries to cool itself in preparation for running or fighting. You may feel sweaty.

So, your body is doing exactly what it has been designed to do.

Now, it is highly unlikely that you will experience a very **REAL** threat too often.

However, your brain doesn't know the difference. It simply reacts as it was designed to do and will create a response.

How do we help our amygdala RELAX?

The great news is, we can put things in place to oversee our own brain.

Some people choose to give their amygdala a name – like 'Brenda' (Cool name heh?)

When we give this part of our brain a name, we can speak directly to it when it fires up the threat response.

When you feel all those physical responses during a period of anxiety, you could try this...

> *"Hey Brenda! Thanks so much for protecting me. It's a false alarm! I actually just realised that I had to give a talk in front of my English class this afternoon.*
> *I'm not in any danger.*
> *Thanks anyway.*
> *I've got this!"*

Or...

> *"Hey Brenda, Great response! Boy you were quick – I almost missed that last step and would have taken a big tumble! False alarm though. I'm all good. Thanks for looking out for me."*

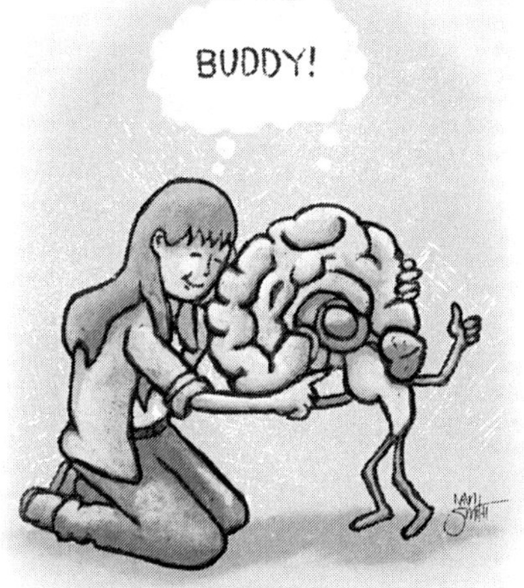

Here are some simple things you can do to calm your body down:

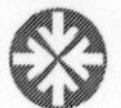 *Bring yourself back to the* **PRESENT**

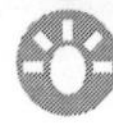 *Make yourself aware of the following using your 5 senses:*

- *What is one thing that you can* **HEAR***?*
- *What is one thing that you can* **SMELL***?*
- *What is one thing you can* **SEE***?*
- *What is one thing you can* **TOUCH***?*
- *What is one thing you can* **TASTE***?*

 **BREATHE** *– To bring your breath back to normal and reduce your heart racing, try this:*

- *Breathe* **IN** *and hold for the count of five*
- *Breathe* **OUT** *slowly for the count of five*
- *Repeat this ten times or longer until you feel calmer*

FOCUS *on something you can control*

Feeling **ANXIOUS** *or* **WORRIED?** *Try some of these:*

- *Read a book*
- *Listen to some relaxing music, podcast, or audiobook*
- *Dance around your room to some tunes*
- *Bounce on a trampoline or do some boxing*
- *Spend time outside in the sunshine*
- *Colour in or draw*
- *Stretching your body*
- *Go for a long walk*
- *Call a friend to chat*
- *Journal your thoughts*
- *Do anything crafty or creative*

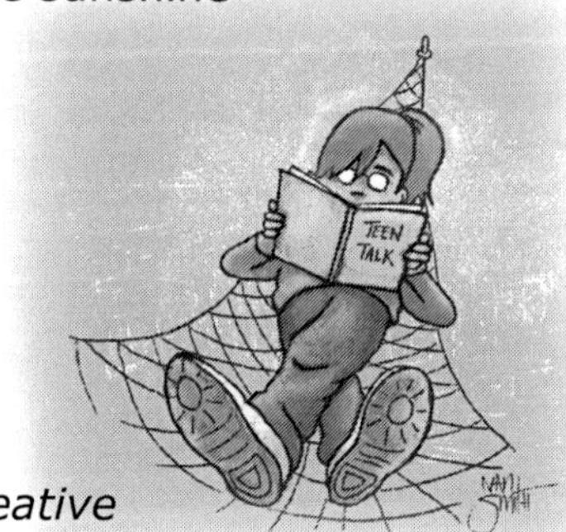

feeling OVERWHELMED?

In our very busy, over-scheduled lives, it can be easy to become overwhelmed when we allow lots of things to build up. I know this from first-hand experience, I get it. We can have loads of expectations that continue to pile in on us. These might include:

- *School assignments*
- *Homework*
- *Part time work*
- *Sports training*
- *Music or Drama practice*
- *Youth group or other social activities*
- *House chores*

Add yours here:

Things that overwhelm me:

Brain dump!

When I begin to feel the overwhelm coming on, I do this practical thing: I take out a piece of paper, some bright pens and I dump everything that feels **BIG** right now and write it down. This way I can **SEE** all the things that I have to get done.

- *Finish my book manuscript*
- *Return 3 phone calls*
- *Clean out my wardrobe*
- *Write article for magazine*
- *Reply to emails*

Break it down!

Your list can be as BIG as you want. Just dump everything that is causing you to feel overwhelmed in that moment. Then I want you to break it down. You can use different colour markers to circle the most urgent things, right down to those of lesser priority.

Do one or two things well

Now, create a plan!
Get out a new piece of paper

- *write the day*
- *write one thing to complete*

Just focus on this one thing today.

Set yourself a reward once you've done it
– e.g. Get out for a walk, eat something delicious, 30 minutes of TV or screen time.

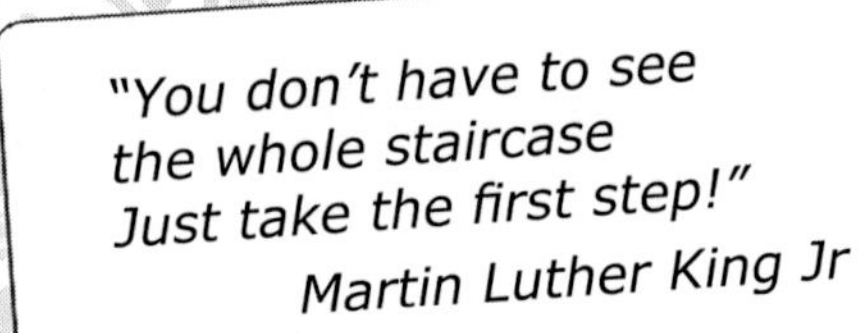

caring for your mental health and wellbeing is just as important as caring for your physical health.

stress soothers

If you are feeling a bit stressed, try some of the following solutions...

EXERCISE! This is great for relieving stress because when you exercise, your body releases its own natural 'feel good' chemicals. It also helps the blood flow better throughout your body, giving it a great boost.

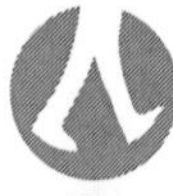

Go for a long **WALK!** (See above.)

Have a couple of **EARLY NIGHTS**. If you are stressed, this could be a sign that your body needs a bit of a rest. Make yourself a warm Milo, grab a good book and read for a little while before having a good, long sleep. You need between eight and 10 hours of sleep per night to feel well rested and stress-free. Make sleep a priority, and your other priorities will fall into place.

EAT WELL! Fill your body with lots of fruit and vegetables. This may sound a bit boring; however, spending a few days giving your body extra minerals and vitamins will help restore you.

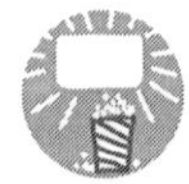

Watch your **FAVOURITE COMEDY** movie.

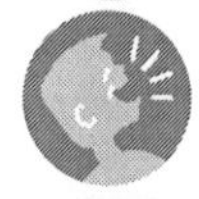

LAUGHTER also releases your body's natural endorphins that help to make you feel better.

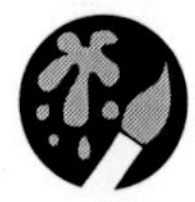

Do something you **LOVE DOING**, e.g.: paint, draw, write, hike, ride, or make something. What is your passion?

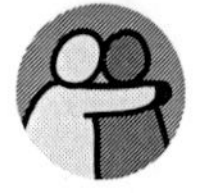

Spend a day out with **FRIENDS**; go shopping, play soccer, hang out together.

Stress

Stress is a common experience for many girls, as you navigate the challenges of growing up, including school, relationships, and future goals. The pressure to succeed academically, socially, and in extracurricular activities can be overwhelming, and can lead to feelings of anxiety, frustration, and even depression.

You may also experience stress due to family conflicts, changes in your living situation, or other external factors beyond your control. While some stress can be beneficial and motivating, too much stress can have negative effects on your physical and mental health.

It's important to recognise when you are feeling stressed and to develop healthy coping strategies, such as exercise, relaxation techniques, talking to a trusted friend or adult, or seeking professional help if needed. By learning to manage stress, you can improve your overall well-being.

Find healthy outlets for dealing with stress – some people exercise or talk with friends. Find what best suits you, and take action.

One big stress indicator is illness, so make sure you take stress seriously and keep a healthy check on yourself.

Stress Indicators:

- *Inability to sleep properly.*
- *Not being able to eat – disinterest in food.*
- *Lack of interest in friends and things that you usually enjoy doing.*
- *Crying often or feeling down in the dumps.*
- *A feeling of being unable to cope.*

If you are struggling with any of the above symptoms for a few weeks, you could very well be struggling with stress. It is important that you talk with your trusted adult: parents, teacher, or school counsellor. It would also be good to visit your local doctor to get a thorough examination.

overcoming perfectionism

Lessons from a recovering perfectionist

This is a chapter for those girls who struggle with **PERFECTIONISM**. Perhaps you relate to this, or you may not. If this doesn't apply to you, feel free to move on from this page. If you can relate, please read on!

The fact that you are holding this book in your hand right now is, in fact, a miracle! Because, like many people – I only want to put something out in the public when I am 100% happy with it – when it is as perfect as it can be. Does this sound familiar?

Maybe you have an assignment due for Science, or an essay for English. You have worked on it for as much time as you have been able to set aside. You check that you have completed each of the assessment points, however you still feel that you just had an extra week, you could make it brilliant. However, you also have a pile of work for other subjects, and to make this assignment perfect, you:

- *Must stay up all night to get it to your version of perfection (which is basically impossible) or*
- *Subject yourself to much more stress and not have the capacity to complete your other assignments well.*

When I work with my secondary students, I encourage them to ask themselves this simple question before they submit a piece of work:

> *"Is this the best I could do, with the time I had to commit to it, and with everything else that may be going on in my world right now?"*

If they can honestly answer yes to this question, I ask them to submit their work. I don't expect perfection from them. I expect the best they can do.

Perfectionism is a common trait among teenagers. You may feel like you need to be perfect in everything you do, whether its to meet high expectations from society, family, or even yourself. However, striving for perfection can lead to feelings of anxiety, depression, and low self-esteem when you fall short of your own ideals. It can also be a roadblock to personal growth and prevent you from trying new things or taking risks.

The good news is that perfectionism is not a fixed trait. You can learn to overcome it and embrace imperfection. Here are some steps:

Identify the roots of your perfectionism

The first step to overcoming perfectionism is to understand where it comes from. It could be from a parent or teacher who always demanded perfection from you, or it could be from your own beliefs and expectations. Try to identify the roots of your perfectionism so you can better understand it and work to overcome it.

Challenge your beliefs

Perfectionism is often driven by unrealistic beliefs and expectations. Challenge these beliefs by asking yourself questions such as, "Is it really necessary to be perfect in everything?" or "What would happen if I let go of this need to be perfect?" This can help you shift your mindset and realise that imperfection is okay.

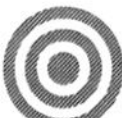

Set realistic goals

One way to overcome perfectionism is to set realistic goals. Instead of setting impossibly high standards, set goals that are achievable and measurable. This will help you feel a sense of accomplishment, and help you learn from any mistakes or failures along the way.

Learn to accept and embrace imperfection

Learning to accept and embrace imperfection is a key step in overcoming perfectionism. Start by recognising that nobody is perfect, and that imperfection is a normal part of the human experience. Practice self-compassion and treat yourself with kindness when you make mistakes.

Think of it this way – if I waited until I thought my manuscript was 100% perfect for this book – you would not be reading it at this moment. It would still be on my laptop. I like to think that 80% great and 100% out there in the bookstores is far better than 100% NOT published.

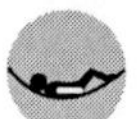

Practice self-care and relaxation

Practising some relaxation techniques such as getting out in nature, going for a walk, exercising, doing things that bring you joy. These are all opportunities to de-stress when the desire to get something 'absolutely perfect' is weighing on you. Try to take a break – stressing about something not being perfect will not make it any better.

Seek support

Overcoming perfectionism can be challenging, and it's important to seek support from friends, a helpful adult in your life, family, or a mental health professional if it is getting in the way of your schoolwork/life. Talking to someone who understands what you're going through can help you feel less alone and can also provide you with helpful strategies.

Finally, I want you to know that I worked really, REALLY hard on this book for you. Is it the very best it could be? Well, to answer that, I would say it is the best I could achieve with the time that I committed to it (which was a LOT!), and the other things in life that I was dealing with over the three years I took to finally send this off to the designers!

Overcoming perfectionism takes time and effort, but it's worth it in the end. By challenging your beliefs, setting realistic goals, embracing imperfection, practicing mindfulness, and seeking support, you can learn to let go of the need to be perfect and embrace your true self. Imperfection is what makes you unique and special, and it's okay to make mistakes and learn from them.

decisions, decisions, decisions...

In your teen years, you'll no doubt be faced with thousands of choices along the way, every day. There'll be choices to make — from what to wear and how to style your hair to whether to hang out with a certain group of girls.

Sometimes, you'll make the right decision. At other times, you'll make the wrong choices and perhaps feel rotten.

The fantastic thing is that we have all been created with an inbuilt mechanism called our ***intuition***, otherwise known as your gut instinct!

Your intuition is a bit like an inner voice or feeling that often lets you know what the right choice to make is. For some people, it feels a bit like a thousand butterflies having a big party in your stomach. At other times, when it is the right decision, it can feel really peaceful and settled — that is your intuition or conscience!

When you are faced with what seems like a difficult choice, try this: Pretend that you have definitely made a decision, one way or another. Now how do you ***feel*** now that you have made that decision? What is your inner voice or gut feeling telling you? If you have made a clear decision, yet you still feel uneasy in your stomach, perhaps you need to re-examine your decision and maybe seek further advice.

Just remember, there will be many, many times that you will make a decision in life and it will turn out to be the wrong one. But that's okay, providing you are not putting yourself or anyone else in danger. These are important learning opportunities.

If in doubt, always ask advice from people you trust — other friends, parents, youth group leaders, teachers or school counsellors. They can often give you helpful advice to help you make the best decision.

inspiring...

'Growing is a lifetime job, and we grow most when we're down in the valleys where the fertiliser is.'

Barbara Johnson

'Every small positive change we make in ourselves pays us in confidence in the future.'

Alice Walker,
American novelist

'Take chances, make mistakes. That's how you grow. Pain nourishes your courage. You have to fail in order to Practise being braver.'

Mary Tyler Moore,
American actress

'Don't judge each day by the harvest you reap but by the seeds that you plant.'

Robert Louis Stevenson

'The rung of a ladder was never meant to rest upon, but only to hold a man's foot long enough to enable him to put the other somewhat higher.'

Thomas Henry Huxley,
Life and letters of Thomas Huxley

'Fall seven times, stand up eight.'

Japanese proverb

' "For I know the plans I have for you," says the Lord. "They are plans for good and not for disaster, to give you a future and hope." '

Jeremiah 29:11
NLT

helpful support

There may be times that you are feeling a bit lost. I want to remind you that you are never alone. I've provided some helpful numbers and websites below that you can utilise at any time.

- **Kids Helpline**
  1800 55 1800
  Free, confidential counselling service available any time of the day or night by phone or webchat.
  www.kidshelpline.com.au

- **Beyond Blue**
  1300 22 4636
  Call or chat online with a counsellor at any time. This Support Service is available 24/7.
  www.beyondblue.org.au

- **headspace**
  1800 650 890
  Online and telephone support service that helps young people who don't feel ready to attend a headspace centre or who prefer to talk about their problems via online chat, email or on the phone.
  www.headspace.org.au

- **Lifeline**
  13 11 44
  www.lifeline.org.au

- **For Online bullying and support**
  www.esafety.gov.au

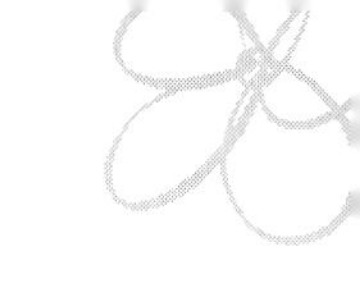

a final word from me

Dear amazing teen girl,

Thanks so much for taking the time to read **Teen Talk — Girl Talk**.

I hope that it has been helpful in answering some of your most pressing questions about growing up, puberty, friendships, body-image and so much more!

I also hope that you've gained some more confidence in navigating these years when reading about other girls' teenage experiences. Remember, being a girl is a precious thing and a privilege.

Never forget that you are an incredible person with amazing qualities, gifts, and talents that need to be shared with the world.

No matter how difficult these years may feel at times, try and remember that everything eventually passes, and you have everything within you to cope with any challenges that come your way.

You have a wonderfully amazing life ahead of you and you are capable of being anything you want to be.

Go get out there and enjoy!

With love,

Sharon x

with thanks

When I initially wrote the Teen Talk series of books for my students, sixteen years ago, I had absolutely NO idea they would go into reprint many times, sell many thousands of copies, and reach so many young people. I am truly humbled and incredibly grateful to be able to speak into the lives of so many teens around the world through the pages of this book.

The original series of this book led me on some amazing adventures and allowed so many new opportunities to come my way that I never dreamt were possible. From appearing regularly on television programs, speaking on radio, writing articles for magazines, and then going on to launch a major conference that now runs Australia-wide – who would have thought?! I have also met some incredible people that came into my life through these new opportunities; many of these have become life-long friends and great supports to me in tough times I've experienced over the past decade.

So, I am incredibly grateful that I made that brave and courageous move all those years ago to step out of my comfort zone and into my courage zone – something I encourage all people that come my way to do, including teens. Because it is in pushing through that initial discomfort and fear, to do something new and challenging, that can lead us to so many new adventures.

I am incredibly thankful for my gorgeous children, now young adult, Josh, and Emily. You guys have loved me and supported me and cheered me on always. I hope that through me living out my dreams and working hard, you can see that it is always worth it. To my mum and dad: I thank you for always being there for me and stepping in when I need extra care and support.

To my amazingly talented graphic designer, Ivan Smith: thank you doesn't seem nearly adequate for all that you do to bring my books to life. Thank you for sharing your talent with the world.

To my wonderful students – both past and present – I am so grateful to you all. You continue to inspire me every day. With particular thanks to my students who so diligently proofread the final pages of this book to ensure it was the best it could be. Thank you for your helpful and honest suggestions. A special thanks to the gorgeous girls who shared their stories in this book.

And to everyone who has supported my work over the past sixteen years, and especially those who have purchased and shared my books so widely – thank you. Your support has enabled me to keep producing these resources.

Sharon x

I'D LOVE TO HEAR FROM YOU!

As you can probably gather, I am a **HUGE FAN** of teenagers.

I always appreciate and value any feedback I receive from my readers.

If any part of this book particularly resonated with you, or you have anything that you think needs to be added to a future edition of this book, feel free to drop me a line. Even if you just want to let me know if this book has impacted you in a positive way. I'd love to hear from you.

You can email me at:

sharon@sharonwitt.com.au

I always try and respond to all my messages

Just be patient if I don't reply immediately ☺.

Sharon x

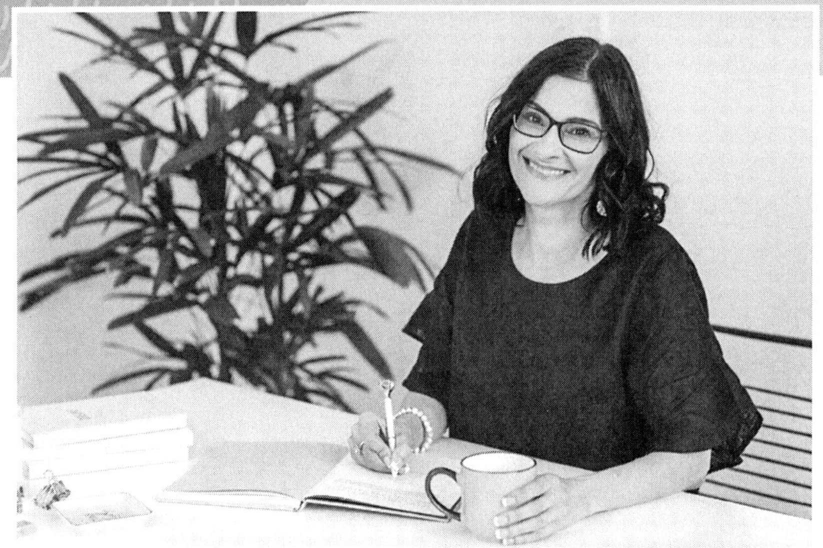

About the author

Sharon Witt has been immersed in the teen world for over three decades in her role as a secondary school teacher, and as an author and presenter to adolescents and their parents around the country.

She is a regular media commentator on issues impacting young people, parenting and educational issues. Sharon is the author of 18 books written for young people to help guide them through many of the issues they face in early years, including the best-selling **Teen Talk**, **Girlwise** and **Wiseguys** series.

Sharon is also the founder of Resilient Kids Conference®, an Australia wide, one-day conference that brings together some of Australia's leading experts on building resilience in young people and their parents.

Her favourite thing is to present to teens in schools and events around the country.

She is mum to two grown adults and resides in Melbourne, Australia.

www.sharonwitt.com.au

My Notes